Caritas in Communion

Theological Foundations of Catholic Health Care

By M. Therese Lysaught, Ph.D.

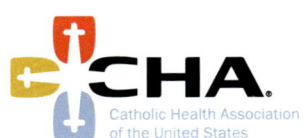

CHA.
Catholic Health Association
of the United States

Library of Congress Cataloging-in-Publication Data
Lysaught, M. Therese
Theological foundations of Catholic health care

Includes a bibliography

1. Catholic health facilities, United States
2. Catholic identity
3. Theology of cooperation

© Copyright 2014 by The Catholic Health Association of the United States
4455 Woodson Road, St. Louis, Mo. 63134-3797

ISBN 978-0-87125-290-6

To order copies or obtain ordering information, please contact CHA
Service Center at **(800) 230-7823**.

Printed in the United States of America.

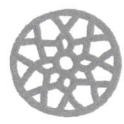

CONTENTS

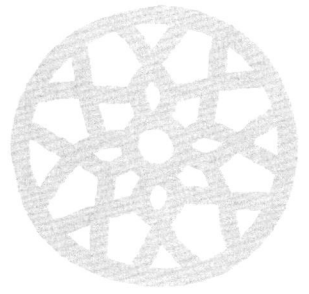

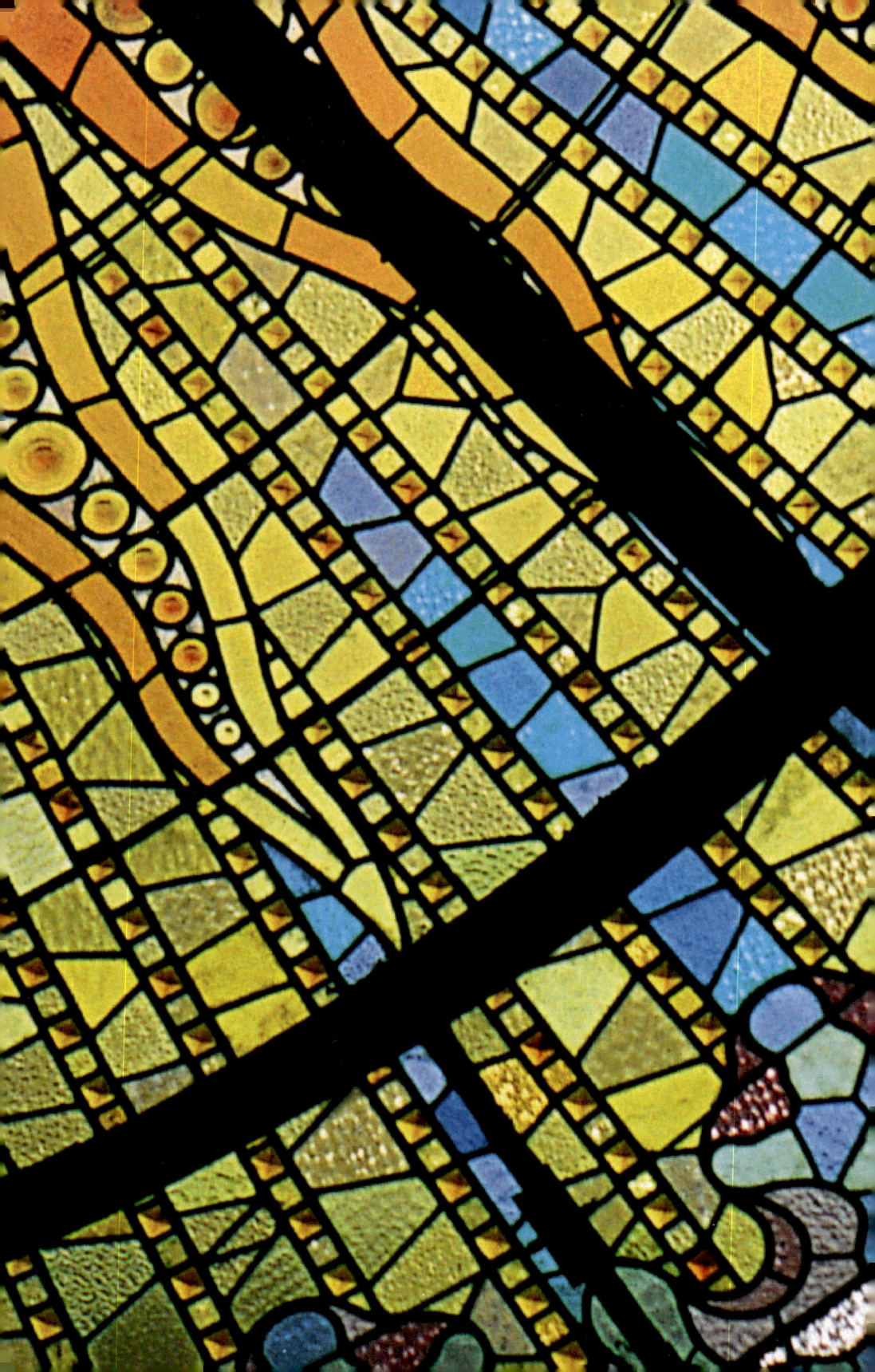

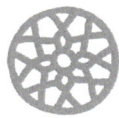

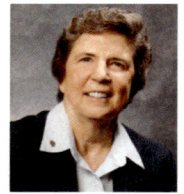The Catholic Health Association will commemorate its one hundredth anniversary in 2015. The motto chosen for CHA in 1915 – *Caritas Christi Urget Nos* (the charity of Christ urges us on) – still expresses CHA's reality, most especially in the midst of a rapidly changing health care environment.

In order to fully address health care changes and its emerging forms, in 2012 CHA's Board of Trustees began a three-year process of discernment to assess CHA's membership criteria. The board requested that the first year's effort (2013) be rooted in theological reflection and articulation of the foundations upon which Catholic health care is grounded. Catholic teaching and principles continually urge the ministry forward even as times change. Moreover, the board hoped that the study document would inform the ministry's thinking about CHA membership criteria — a topic that will be addressed in 2014 and 2015.

Fortuitously, during 2013, M. Therese Lysaught, Ph.D. served as visiting scholar at CHA. Dr. Lysaught is professor at Loyola University, Chicago, in both the Institute of Pastoral Studies and the Neiswanger Institute for Bioethics and Health Policy. She led wide consultations with CHA members, including board members, sponsors, mission leaders, theologians and ethicists about their experience and convictions regarding Catholic health care. Dr. Lysaught's purpose was to describe (rather than define) what Catholic health care is in order to shape what it continues to become. Furthermore, throughout the study, Dr. Lysaught examined newly emerging forms of Catholic health care to discern which ones best embody the Good News of the Gospel and enable Catholic ministries to incarnate God's grace in today's world.

The study we share with you is a snapshot in time. We at CHA hope that it will stimulate study, conversation and communal evaluations that are deeply rooted in our faith tradition. May it feed your spirit and inspire your work.

Sister Carol Keehan

Sister Carol Keehan, DC
President and Chief Executive Officer
Catholic Health Association of the United States

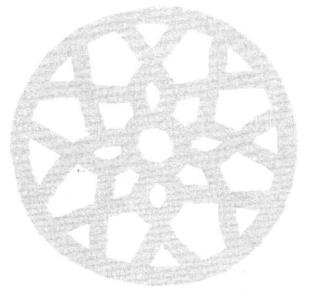

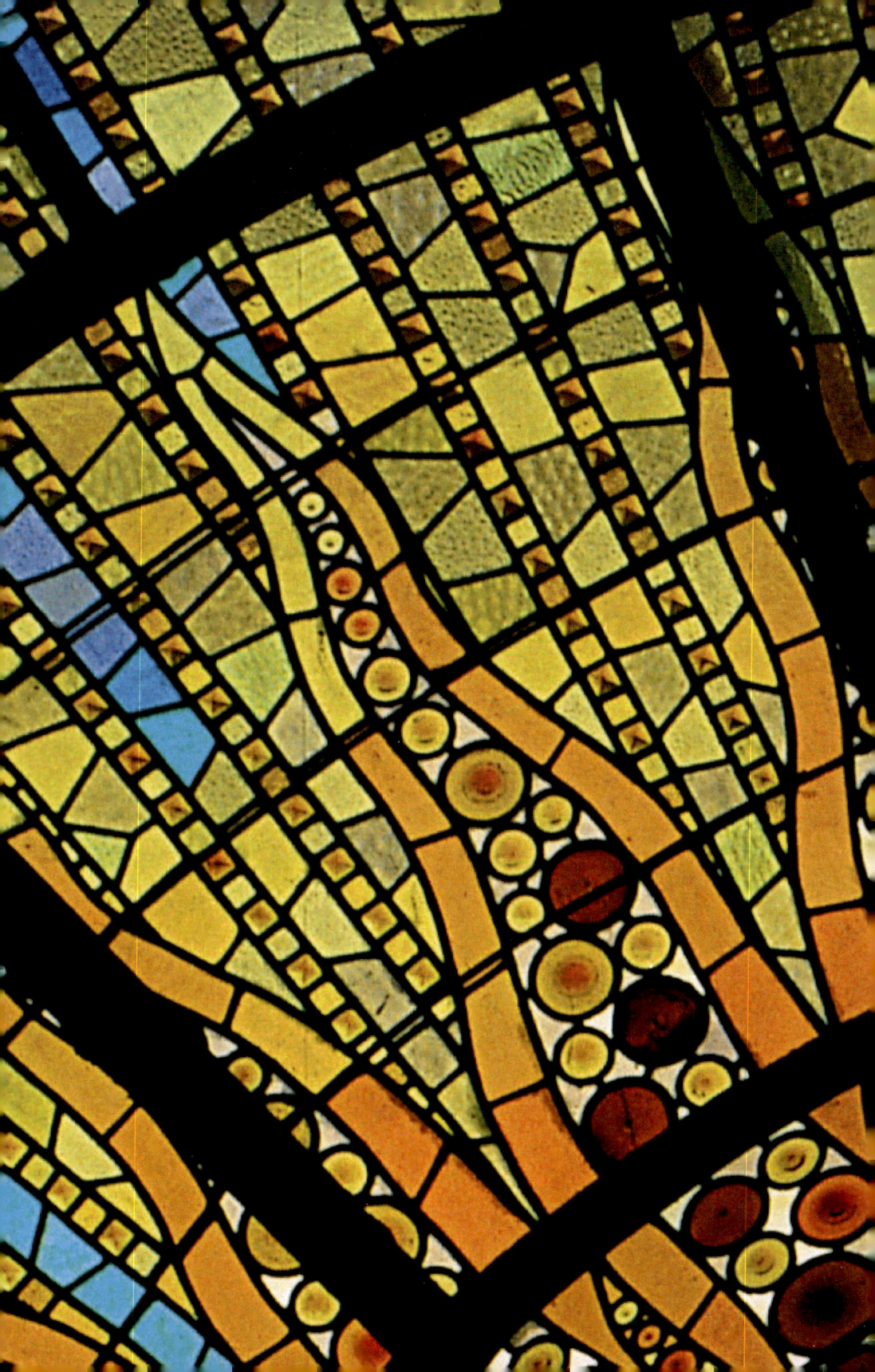

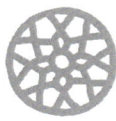

I. INTRODUCTION

CATHOLIC HEALTH CARE ONCE AGAIN FINDS itself working within a changing landscape. Change has been the constant companion of Catholic health care in the United States since the Ursuline Sisters in New Orleans opened the first privately owned Catholic hospital in 1728. From the establishment of Catholic hospitals amidst epidemics, wars, urban immigrant poverty and frontier chaos in the latter half of the 19TH century, to the medical modernization and professionalization of Catholic hospitals in the early 20TH century, to growth spurred by the Hill-Burton Act and Medicaid/Medicare funding in the 1950s and 1960s, to the move toward Catholic systems in the 1970s, 1980s and 1990s—the women and men who founded, worked, led, built, and continually transformed the significant infrastructure that is now U.S. Catholic health care met shifts in medicine and the market with insight, innovation and integrity made possible by grace.[1]

Most of these changes were simply changes of scale—moving from 12 beds to 200; moving from charitable donations and voluntary payers

---

1. For the most comprehensive history of Catholic health care in the United States, see Christopher J. Kauffman, *Ministry and Meaning: A Religious History of Catholic Health Care in the United States* (New York: Crossroad Publishing Company, 1995).

to significant amounts of government funding; moving from stand-alone Catholic hospitals to collaborative Catholic health systems. Recent developments seem more fundamental. They are not simply a matter of scope and scale. Some systems have decided to forgo formal recognition by the diocesan bishop. Other Catholic hospitals or systems have adopted for-profit corporate structures. Others are considering variations on these new models. Clinical integration networks and accountable care organizations, which reconceptualize medicine away from acute-level, hospital-focused, fee-for-service care to more clinic or community-centered population health management approaches, shift the landscape in yet another way.

Over two decades ago, Joseph Cardinal Bernardin, named the key tension raised by these shifts. In speaking of "Catholic Institutions and Their Identity," he recognized that:

> Catholic colleges and universities, health care institutions and social service agencies already live with one foot firmly planted in the Catholic Church and the other in our pluralistic society….[Thus, they] face a common dilemma. The bishop and diocese at times may consider them too secular, too influenced by government, too involved with business concepts. The public, on the other hand, often considers them too religious, too sectarian. As a result, they find themselves sandwiched between the church and the public, trying to please both groups….A mixed model of identity will prevail in the future, not a strictly denominational or secular one.[2]

Cardinal Bernardin's words now appear quite prophetic. Mixed models of identity are clearly emerging.

These mixed models raise new questions for Catholic health care. What does it mean to be a Catholic institution? Can an organization

---

2. Joseph Bernardin, "Catholic Institutions and Their Identity," *Origins* 21, no. 2 (May 23, 1991): 33-6.

maintain its Catholic identity if it is owned and/or managed by an other-than-Catholic organization? If so, how? How might for-profit status impact Catholic identity? Is for-profit culture compatible with Catholic culture or are they mutually exclusive?

For the Catholic Health Association (CHA), these developments raise a pragmatic issue. The criteria for CHA membership, crafted in the 1960s and reaffirmed via a membership discernment process in 1993, are quite straightforward. To be a member of CHA, a hospital or system must:

1. Be recognized as Catholic by the diocesan bishop
2. Be located in the U.S.
3. Promote or foster the values of the Catholic health ministry
4. Embrace and support the mission and purposes of the Association
5. Be a not-for-profit entity.

These criteria are well grounded in the tradition and experience of Catholic health care. Yet with the recent developments, some systems or hospitals that have adopted these new configurations no longer qualify for CHA membership.

This conundrum called CHA to initiate a process of discernment around its membership criteria. CHA, however, is simply the public voice of Catholic health care. Therefore, this discernment process is, in reality, discernment by Catholic health care as a whole. CHA has outlined a three-year timetable for this process. Year one (2013) has engaged in a necessary first step: to clearly articulate the *theological foundations* of Catholic health care. During year two (2014), the CHA Board of Trustees and the membership as a whole will reflect on the *lived experience* of Catholic health care, especially of those who have adopted these new models, in light of these theological foundations. During year three (2015), they will revisit the CHA membership criteria in light of these foundations and the experiences.

The end result will be a decision regarding the CHA membership criteria taken by Catholic health care as a whole.

This study presents the fruits of the first year of this process: an account of the *theological foundations* of Catholic health care. The process took as its commission the question: *What are the theological questions and analyses that might help inform our discussions about membership?* Toward that end, the study has examined three main issues: (1) the theological foundations of *Catholic identity* in Catholic health care; (2) the theological foundations of *the principle of moral cooperation* insofar as it is the primary framework used to address partnerships between Catholic, faith-based, and secular organizations; and (3) the theological foundations of Catholic economic thought as they relate to the question of *for-profit corporate status.*

These analyses have produced a substantive, robust account of those *theological* commitments that ground the work of the Catholic health care ministry. To be clear, this study is *not* doing a number of things. It is not making specific recommendations about how health care organizations might concretely embody Catholic identity. It is not making specific recommendations regarding behaviors that embody Catholic identity or how it might be assessed. It is not outlining ways that Catholic identity might evolve in the future based on its interface with these new realities. It is not making specific recommendations regarding membership criteria. These are tasks for the next two years of the discernment process—and beyond.

1.1 A NOTE ON METHOD

This discernment is a process for Catholic health care by Catholic health care. As such, this first phase of discernment has employed an inductive, dialogical method. The process began with interviews with board members, mission leaders, sponsors and others by the consulting firm Noblis of Falls Church, Va. In these interviews, key stakeholders in Catholic health care were asked: What is essential for Catholic health care to be Catholic? What are your worries or concerns?

The findings from these interviews provided helpful points of orientation for subsequent research. An interdisciplinary group of theologians from the academy and health care was convened. The group gave initial feedback on the project as a whole and assisted with resources and feedback as the project moved forward. In addition to CHA staff, the working group included:

Rev. Albino Barrera, OP, Ph.D., Providence (R.I.) College (ethics and economics)

Rev. Steven Bevans, SVD, Ph.D., Catholic Theological Union, Chicago (mission)

Charles Clark, Ph.D., St. John's University, New York (economics)

Clarke E. Cochran, Ph.D., St. Joseph Health, Irvine, Calif. (public policy)

Shannon Dwyer, JD, St. Joseph Health, Irvine, Calif. (legal)

Sr. Doris Gottemoeller, RSM, Ph.D., Catholic Health Partners, Cincinnati (ecclesiology)

John Hardt, Ph.D., Loyola University Chicago (ethics)

M. Therese Lysaught, Ph.D., Loyola University Chicago (formerly of Marquette University, Milwaukee) (theological ethics)

Rev. Richard Sparks, CSP, Ph.D., St. Mary's University, San Francisco (ethics)

Sr. Marlene Weisenbeck, FSPA, Ph.D., JCL, Franciscan
Sisters of Perpetual Adoration, La Crosse, Wis. (canon law)

Susan Wood, SCL, Ph.D., Marquette University, Milwaukee
(ecclesiology)

Daniel Finn, Ph.D., St. John's University, Collegeville, Minn.
(ethics and economics)

Based on the input of the working group, an extensive bibliography
on the questions of Catholic identity, the principle of moral
cooperation, and profit-status was compiled and researched. This
bibliography drew primarily from the literature on Catholic health
care but also from the ongoing debate on Catholic identity in
Catholic higher education that has continued since Pope John Paul
II issued *Ex Corde Ecclesiae* in 1990. The literature of Catholic health
care was given priority in this study in order to proceed as inductively
as possible—the project sought to begin with the voices, wisdom and
lived experience of leaders and theologians who work in Catholic
health care, so as to ground the findings of this project in the realities
of Catholic health care. It also gave priority to the writings of the
Catholic social tradition, particularly the writings of Popes John Paul
and Benedict XVI. Initial findings from this research were presented
to CHA staff, to members of the working group, and to annual
gatherings of system mission leaders, sponsors, theologians and
ethicists for feedback and input. The paper was revised repeatedly in
light of that feedback. In short, the method for this study has been an
iterative process of listening, study, analysis and revision.[3]

---

3. The Working Group—and the many groups that were consulted in the process—were essential
in beating much of the chaff out of earlier versions of this document. Because of the involvement of
so many persons in this final product, the document occasionally uses the plural "we" when referring
to authorship.

1.2 SUMMARY OF FINDINGS

The church, Catholic health care and the world at large are in a time of change, ferment and transformation. In the midst of this ferment, Pope Benedict called Catholics to engage the world in as-yet-unimagined ways. In *Caritas in Veritate,* he identifies the urgent need for new forms of commitment, engagement, cooperation (§21-24) and for "a profoundly new way of understanding the business enterprise" (§40).

Catholic health care has already embraced this call. Yet it may be that not all new forms are equal. The challenge is to discern which new forms and new ways best embody the unchanging Good News of the Gospel and enable Catholics concretely to incarnate God's grace in this new context, in and for the sake of the world.

A first step in addressing this challenge is to step back from the whirlwind of change and to reflect anew on the essentials of the Gospel and the Catholic tradition. What is at the heart of the Gospel that these new forms must necessarily carry forward? Where do we find warrants (sound reasons) in our tradition for innovative structures? How might new structures lift up elements of the Gospel or church that had been constrained by previous forms and unleash God's grace in new and powerful ways? How might new structures, alternatively, impede the Spirit's ability to work in the world?

As we plumb the tradition for its insights on Catholic identity, cooperation and the for-profit question, this study seeks to lift up key elements of the rich, vibrant Catholic tradition that underlies the powerful work of Catholic health care. It brings into the conversation concrete proposals about new forms of engagement, cooperation and enterprise. And it identifies new questions, areas that need further empirical research, conceptual analysis and theological development.

At the heart of all these questions—identity, cooperation, economics—we find a consistent conviction: that the theological center of all that we are and do as Catholics is *caritas* in communion, God's love manifest in communion. The challenge for Catholic health care is to discern which structures best enable the church— and particularly lay persons—to carry on the tradition of *caritas* in communion initiated by God in creation, given to Christians and the church through Christ, and continued in our context through the charisms of the founders of Catholic health care. Such *caritas* has a particular shape—it is sacramental and ecclesial, ministerial and evangelical. It is necessarily characterized by dialogue, mutuality, communion, solidarity, relation and a recognition of all persons as members of God's human family. It translates, in the business context, into the principle of gratuitousness and particular care for those who do the work of Catholic health care. In other words, the fruit of *caritas* in the world is always communion.

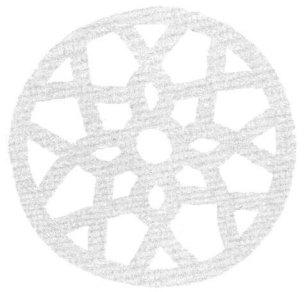

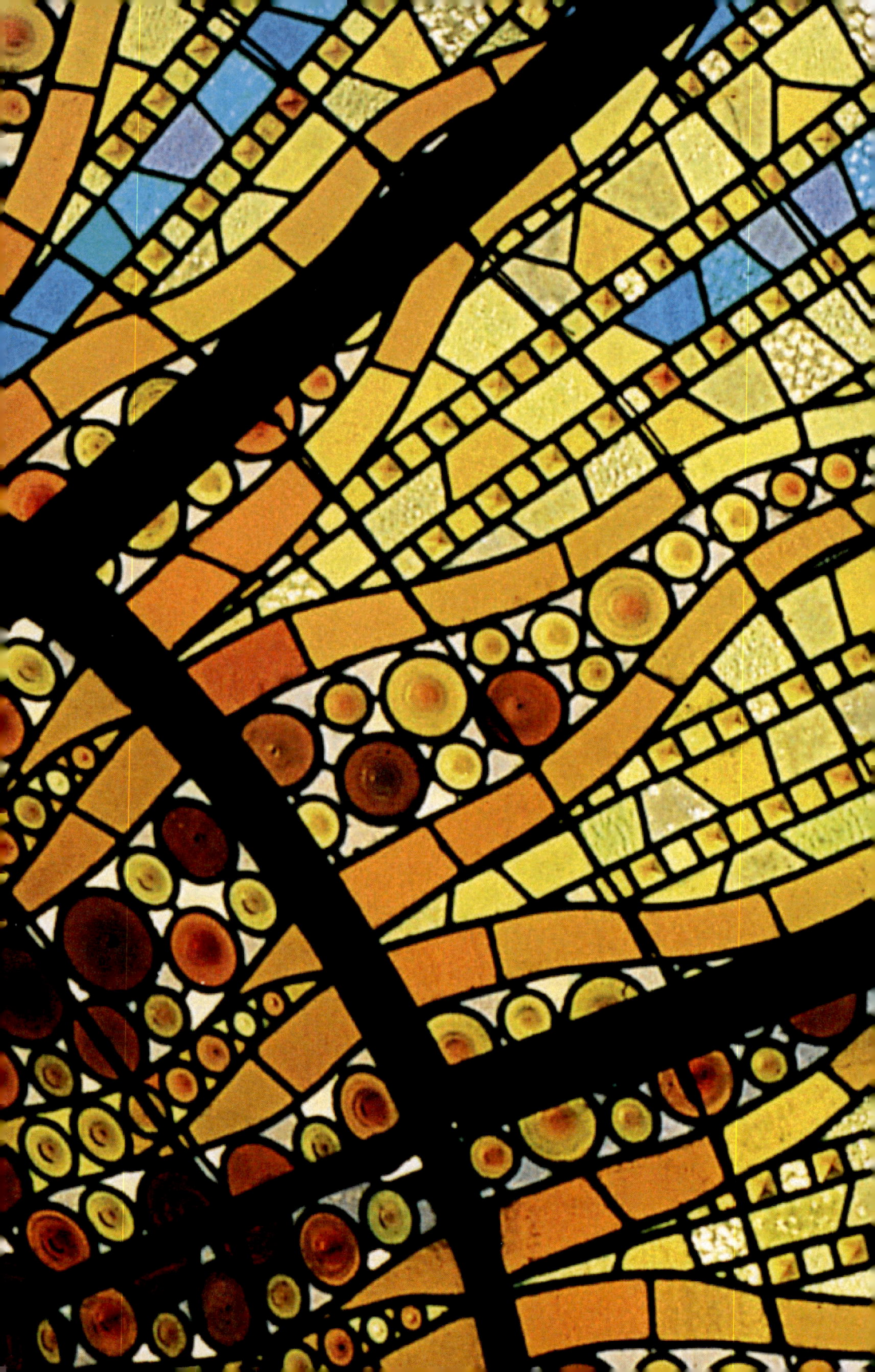

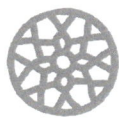

II. EMERGING MODELS AND
CURRENT DEVELOPMENTS

W HAT ARE THE EMERGING ORGANIZATIONAL models that are reshaping Catholic health care? The field is a moving target, and variations will likely continue to evolve. However, regardless of the exact form of any new model, the following questions provide a framework for analyzing the ways any new model interfaces with traditional dimensions of Catholic health care organizations:

1. What is the religious identity of the parent organization? …of the individual hospitals?[4]

2. What is the for-profit/not-for-profit status of the parent organization…of the individual hospitals?

3. How are the relationships between Catholic and other-than-Catholic components of the system mediated or structured?

4. What is the relationship between the system, hospitals, and diocesan bishops?

---

4. The term "hospitals" is used in this study in a generic sense to include all health care entities such as hospitals, long-term care facilities, clinics, etc.

5.   What is the role of the sponsors?

Set forth below are some examples of new models that have emerged thus far. These models are schematic and are described with attention to these questions.

A FOR-PROFIT VENTURE FUND ACQUIRES A CATHOLIC SYSTEM

A first model is one in which a secular for-profit venture fund acquires a Catholic system. As part of the transaction, the system and its hospitals become for-profit entities. The diocesan bishop, however, continues to recognize the systems' hospitals as Catholic. A contractual "stewardship agreement" might be entered into, whereby the hospitals would continue to abide by the *Ethical and Religious Directives for Catholic Health Care Services (Directives),* staff mission and pastoral care departments, allow the sacraments to be provided and/or specify guidelines for uncompensated care.

A CATHOLIC SYSTEM FORMS A FOR-PROFIT VENTURE FUND TO ACQUIRE CATHOLIC HOSPITALS

A second model involves the creation of a new joint venture relationship between a not-for-profit Catholic health system and a private equity firm. The new venture seeks to acquire financially strapped Catholic hospitals and health systems and convert them to for-profit status, while retaining their Catholic identity. The Catholic system is a minority partner in the arrangement, but retains sole authority to set the charity and community benefit policies which will be consistent with those followed in the not-for-profit hospitals operated by the system. The for-profit hospitals will continue to follow the *Directives* and be recognized by their diocesan bishops as Catholic. The system's sponsors will sponsor the joint venture, which will be officially recognized as Catholic.

A FOR-PROFIT HEALTH CARE SYSTEM ACQUIRES A CATHOLIC HOSPITAL

In another model that emerged in the 1990s, publicly traded for-profit health care corporations acquired individual Catholic hospitals. In these arrangements, the parent system is secular. Both the parent company and the hospitals are for-profit. The Catholic hospitals may attempt to retain their Catholic identity in different ways. Some may voluntarily choose to continue to follow the *Directives* and other Catholic practices without involvement of sponsors or official recognition of the hospital as Catholic by the diocesan bishop. In other situations, the diocesan bishop may continue to recognize the hospital as Catholic. Sponsors may not technically be involved in sponsorship but instead limit their role to mission/pastoral care. In these situations, there tend to be only a few Catholic hospitals in a much larger network of primarily community hospitals.

A CATHOLIC SYSTEM REORGANIZES INTO AN OTHER-THAN-CATHOLIC PARENT STRUCTURE

In another variation, a Catholic system which owns and operates both Catholic and other-than- Catholic hospitals, decides—in consultation with the diocesan bishops with whom it had been in relationship—to restructure its governance as follows: (a) the system and all hospitals would remain not-for-profit; (b) the parent organization itself would no longer be officially recognized as Catholic by diocesan bishops; and (c) the individual hospitals would retain their respective identities as either Catholic or other-than-Catholic. The Catholic hospitals would continue to follow the *Directives* and the other-than-Catholic hospitals would continue to operate under a shared Statement of Common Values. The Catholic hospitals would continue to be recognized as official Catholic ministries by their diocesan bishops. The sponsors may no longer have an official role in the parent organization, but would have a defined set of responsibilities with regard to subcommittees of the parent board and with regard to the Catholic hospitals.

A CATHOLIC/ OTHER-THAN-CATHOLIC AFFILIATION

In another type of affiliation, a Catholic system enters into an affiliation with an other-than-Catholic system through the creation of a "mirror" governance and management structure—two boards and two senior management teams, comprised of the same people, who alternately function as such for the Catholic and other-than-Catholic parts of the system. Each system keeps its name, previous identity and not-for-profit status. The Catholic hospitals remain in relationship with their diocesan bishops and sponsors.

A SECULAR NOT-FOR-PROFIT SYSTEM ACQUIRES A CATHOLIC HOSPITAL

In certain cases, secular, not-for-profit systems have acquired Catholic hospitals. Here the parent organization is secular, the Catholic hospital is Catholic; both are not-for-profit. The Catholic hospital remains in relationship with its diocesan bishop and, in some cases, the sponsors.

Most of these models have emerged quite recently—since 2010. The landscape is still evolving. Some of the models outlined above may prove unworkable and be dissolved. Other new models or variations on the above may well emerge that will raise new questions. At this time, however, some current developments can be identified.

    First, Catholic hospitals and systems are entering into arrangements in which the parent organization is officially other-than-Catholic.

    Second, for-profit or not-for-profit status for the parent structure and hospitals is mostly consistent throughout the structures.

Third, with only a few exceptions, the Catholic hospitals remain in relationship with their diocesan bishops.

Fourth, with only a few exceptions, the Catholic hospitals remain in relationship with their sponsors, but rather than operating at the board level, the role of the sponsors is now more varied, being located at different places in the hospital setting (e.g., mission, pastoral care) or on the organizational chart.

Fifth, in almost every case, the emergence of a new model is motivated by factors very specific to the system's context— financial, geographical, ecclesial.

QUESTIONS FOR REFLECTION AND DISCUSSION

1. What is at the heart of the Gospel that we are responsible to carry forward?

2. At the heart of all these questions … we find a consistent conviction: that the theological center of all that we are and do as Catholics is … God's love manifest in communion. How is *caritas* in communion expressed in the present structures of Catholic health care?

3. How might new structures open up possibilities for God's grace to be unleashed in ways that have been constrained by previous forms?

4. How might we identify elements in the new structures that could impede the Spirit's ability to work in the world?

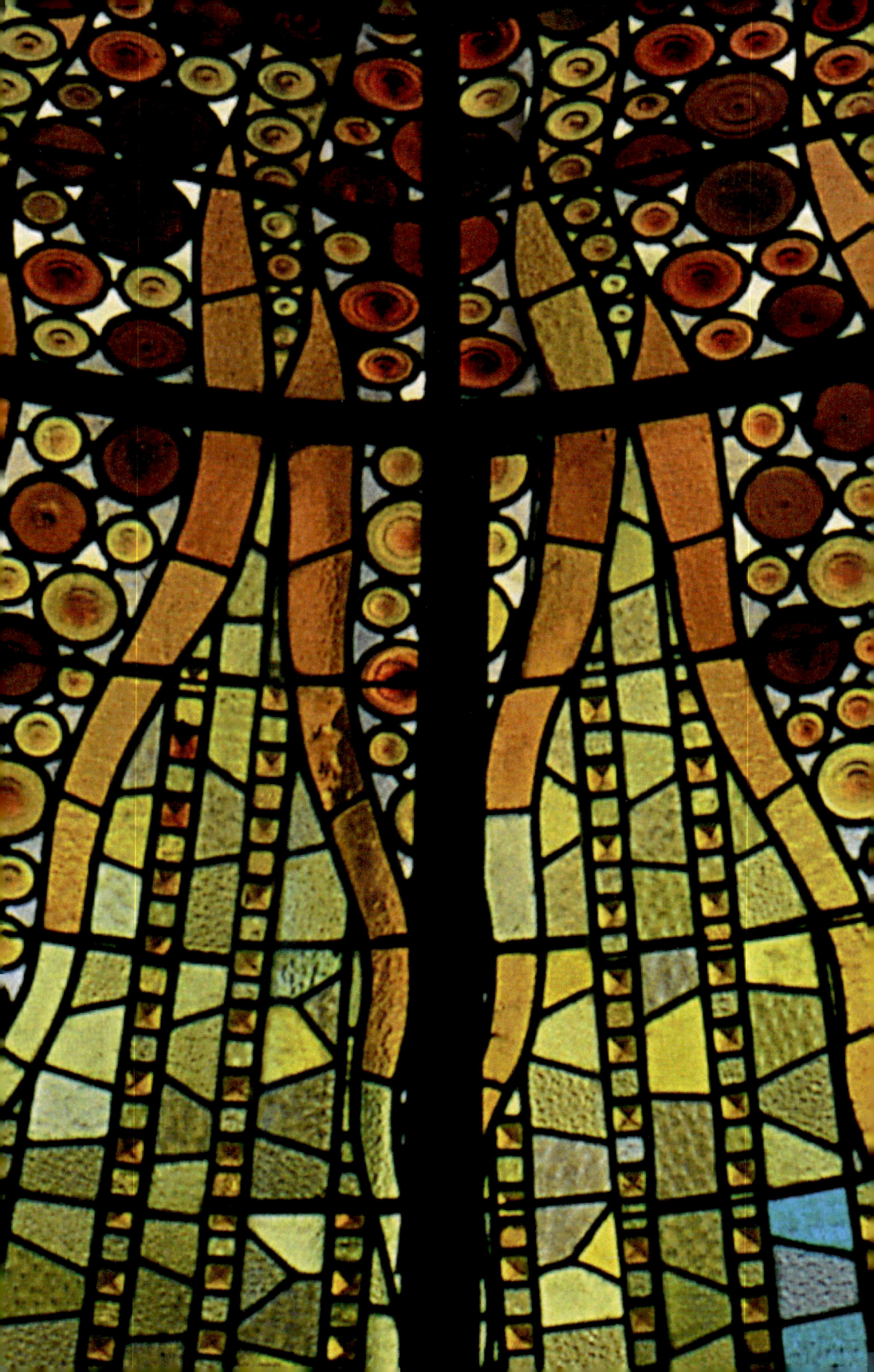

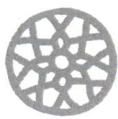

III. THEOLOGICAL FOUNDATIONS OF

CATHOLIC IDENTITY

THE DEVELOPMENTS OUTLINED IN PART II demonstrate the significant efforts being taken by Catholic health care organizations to envision new ways to maintain their Catholic identity. Steps include remaining in relationship with the diocesan bishop and the sponsors and continuing to follow the *Directives*, to offer strong pastoral care and mission services, to offer the sacraments, and to provide a significant level of charity care and community benefit. Are all these elements necessary for an institution to identify as Catholic? Are they sufficient? Might different actions be taken that would embody and further Catholic identity? Is one element sufficient to publically identify as Catholic (for example, approval from the diocesan bishop or a strong commitment to charity care) or is absence of one step sufficient to erase Catholic identity?

These are not new questions. Since the early 1970s, Catholic health care has had a lively debate about Catholic identity. The literature is rich in lived-wisdom on characteristics of Catholic identity. Lists of key characteristics range in length from one[5] to 13.[6] Commentators

---

5. Brian O'Toole, "The Hallmark of Catholic Identity," *Health Progress* 89, no. 3 (May-June 2008): 46, 51, 84.

6. Richard M. Haughian, "A Shared Vision of the Future," *Health Progress* 85, no. 3 (May-June 2004): 45-9.

focus on organizational structures, values, principles, beliefs, behaviors, doctrinal criteria and canonical criteria, in various combinations.

The landscape, in other words, is rich and varied. In addition, Catholic health care itself is rich and varied. There is no such thing as "generic" Catholic health care. As a work of God's grace in the world, Catholic health care incarnates the Gospel in a multifaceted way. Different hospitals and systems embody different facets of the Gospel, following their founders' charisms as they are incarnated in their particular social locations.

The task of this study is to clarify the *theological foundations* of this multifaceted landscape. Such foundations will assist Catholic health care as it continues to discern how hospitals and systems can maintain Catholic identity in these new configurations. Rather than articulating another set of characteristics or a template for assessment, this section asks: what theological grounding underlies the various characteristics of Catholic identity? What theological commitments do the various actions, behaviors, characteristics or elements seek to express in action? By identifying the theological foundations of Catholic identity for Catholic health care, CHA and its members will be able to more clearly articulate which actions or elements are essential for Catholic identity or alternative ways that Catholic identity might faithfully be embodied.

The varied ways of embodying Catholic identity and the diversity of charisms incarnate in Catholic health care reflects the rich and endlessly creative nature of the work of the Trinitarian God in the world. Consequently, an adequate theological foundation for Catholic identity is necessarily multi-layered. At the heart of this foundation we find *caritas,* God's essential nature.[7] God's *caritas* is

---

7. As will be discussed further below, the word *caritas* is often translated as " love" or "charity." But these latter terms have lost the complex theological and practical meanings they once had. Therefore, in this document the word *caritas* is used in order to challenge preconceived notions of "charity" and to broaden our imaginations regarding what *caritas* means in the practice of health care.

manifest in, with and through Jesus and the Spirit—the Trinitarian communion. From this communion emerges a sacramental *caritas-*shaped church, a communion from which baptized Catholics bring *caritas* into the world through ministry and witness to the faith. This *caritas* is vibrantly displayed through the richly diverse work of the founders of our Catholic health systems and the ways in which they have lived the principles of Catholic social thought, key manifestations of God's *caritas* in communion with the world.

3.1 IDENTITY: A CONTEXT

Before turning to Catholic identity itself, let us situate the question in some context. What is the history of our question? What do we mean by "identity"? Four brief observations are pertinent.

First, the question of "Catholic identity" for Catholic institutions is both old and new. University of Notre Dame historian Philip Gleason, Ph.D., captures our current question well in his aptly-titled article: "What Made Catholic Identity a Problem?"[8] Prior to the 1950s, Gleason finds, the "problem" of Catholic identity did not really exist. The Catholic identity of Catholic institutions was largely a given. Catholics and others were confident that Catholics were self-consciously "different"—with distinctive religious beliefs and practices, and that distinctive Catholic institutions were appropriate and important.

This secure sense of Catholic identity begins to erode in the 1950s—prior to the Second Vatican Council, importantly—due to a number of broader societal trends. These included the social assimilation of Catholics into American culture after the Second World War; increases in government funding for social, educational and health

---

8. Philip Gleason, "What Made Catholic Identity a Problem?" (Marianist award lecture, University of Dayton, Dayton, Ohio, 1994). See also Charles E. Curran, "The Catholic Identity of Catholic Institutions," *Theological Studies* 58 (March 1997): 90-108; and Anne M. Clifford, "Identity and Vision at Catholic Colleges and Universities," *Horizons* 35, no. 2 (Fall 2008): 355-70.

care initiatives (such as the GI Bill and the Hill-Burton Act) which spurred tremendous growth of Catholic institutions and increased professionalization of disciplines and state licensing, which Catholic professionals enthusiastically embraced. These forces met Vatican II and the national cultural crises of the 1960s, and, from there forward, Catholic identity becomes a "problem." Catholics and their institutions are no longer clear on what makes them distinctive or whether there should be a "distinctively" Catholic approach to health care or higher education. It is at this point—the early 1970s—that the issue of Catholic identity as a question or problem enters the Catholic health care literature.

Yet, while the question of Catholic identity has been debated for 50 years, within the life of the church, this is a very short time. Therefore, in many ways, it is a new theological question.

Second, what do we mean by identity? Identity is a complex term. As it draws on different disciplines, different facets of the term emerge, potentially pointing in opposite directions. The phrase "Catholic identity" often tilts toward some sort of center or foundation. Here "identity"concerns intrinsic characteristics of a person or institution, characteristics that are consistent over time, that are perceivable by others, that distinguishes a person or institution from some and connects them to others. Identity allows one to "identify" with others, to find points of commonality and unity.[9]

At the same time, these more intrinsic, foundational and communal notions of identity co-exist in the U.S. culture with more psychological or developmental meanings. Here identity has a more individualistic sense, indicating that which makes a person or institution unique. Instead of being stable or unitary, identity is something that emerges over time in response to life experiences, personal interactions and environmental influences.

---

9. This definition draws from the *Oxford English Dictionary* online, oed.com, accessed December 18, 2012, "Identity."

Both senses of identity are important for this study. The question of the *theological foundations* of Catholic health care seeks to discern those intrinsic characteristics shared by all who claim the word "Catholic." What is the common core of *Catholic* health care? What are the indispensable characteristics? Yet clearly, persons and institutions embody multiple identities simultaneously. These multiple identities are lived in the world, amidst persons and institutions with other identities. Living one's identity, thus, is a process of constant negotiation, discerning what it means to live one's core characteristics in this particular place at this particular time. As one does so, core characteristics may develop more fully, with more depth; certain aspects may become nuanced or softened; one may integrate new components into one's identity. And what was once considered core or indispensable may change; for example, up until the 1960s, a seemingly non-negotiable facet of Catholic identity was "no meat on Fridays."

Third, this both/and sense of identity is deeply embedded in the Catholic tradition. The Christian life is understood as a pilgrimage, a journey in which we grow in virtue and holiness. Such growth necessarily emerges in response to particular persons and situations. Dallas Bishop Kevin Farrell in an important address entitled "What Does It Mean To Be Catholic Enough?" details the rich and varied ways that individuals, religious communities, theologians and church leaders have embodied Catholic identity over the past 2,000 years of "Catholic moments." For Bishop Farrell, Catholic identity means:

> …taking very seriously the characteristically Catholic integration of official church teaching, other voices in this theological tradition, our liturgical and sacramental traditions and practices, the variety of spiritualities and prayer forms that it has encouraged and fostered as well as its artistic and aesthetic accomplishments, again with a rich variety reflecting the people and the needs of the church in any and every age.[10]

---

10. Kevin J. Farrell, "What Does It Mean To Be Catholic Enough?" *Origins* 39, no. 11 (August 13, 2009): 189-91.

A humble appreciation of our history reminds us that we are called to bring God's creative grace to each new moment. Therefore, Catholic identity cannot be something fixed or complete. As Bishop Farrell notes, "No theologian or professor or pope has ever had or ever will have all the answers to what it means to be authentically and fully Catholic."[11]

The embeddedness of Catholics and Catholic health care in the particulars of "every age" generates dynamism and concern. Prominent figures such as Catholic health care ethicist Jack Glaser, STD, and Jesuit moral theologian Richard McCormick, STD, became increasingly concerned about the ability of Catholic health care to maintain its identities in the midst of contemporary social, financial and medical systems.[12] McCormick worried that these factors might even make "mission impossible." Others, such as Clarke Cochran, Ph.D. (who is both a political scientist and mission leader), are less despairing. Using the metaphor of "borderlands" to describe the social context of Catholic institutions *vis a vis* U.S. culture, he uses the word "mestizaje" to capture the ways in which "multiple cultures, practices, institutions or authorities meet, not abstractly but in a fully embodied way" and mutually shape each other.[13]

Finally, a robust identity will be perceptible to others. The question of identity is at heart a question of integrity: how do our actions reflect or embody our identity? One might ask: *Who do we say we are?* in order that we might discern *Who are we called to be?* so that we can answer the question *What ought we to do in this situation?*[14] This understanding of integrity reflects the both/and notion of identity stated earlier. Integrity grounds us in a foundational set of characteristics but it also is dynamic, moving us toward an ever fuller

---

11. Farrell.

12. John W. Glaser and Brian B. Glaser, "Systemic Reform Is Vital to Our Ministry," *Health Progress* 83, no. 3 (May-June 2002): 16-9; and Richard A. McCormick, "The Catholic Hospital Today: Mission Impossible?" *Origins* (March 16, 1995): 648-53.

13. Clarke E. Cochran, "Catholic Healthcare in the Public Square: Tension on the Frontier." In *Handbook of Bioethics and Religion,* edited by David Guinn (New York: Oxford University Press, 2006), p. 404.

embodiment of an identity. How we move forward will be shaped by the particulars of where we find ourselves, by the pragmatic limits of possibility in our context. Therefore, there is no one set of actions that can be spelled out in advance. Rather, one's identity can be lived with integrity in a diversity of ways.

While the question of integrity enables us to discern how to move forward, it also challenges us to self-assessment. For our actions necessarily reflect and embody what we believe. Thus, we might ask: *who do our actions say that we are?* Are our actions or behaviors at odds with our stated identity as Catholic? Do our institutions act in such a way, for example, to value profits over persons or to place competition for market share over collaboration for the common good?

In living identity with integrity, Catholic health care *will* be distinctive. It will exercise witness and leadership regarding how health care can be practiced differently. And although the ways of living identity with integrity will necessarily be shaped by context, such actions will *connect* Catholic institutions with others who claim the same identity.

3.2 CATHOLIC IDENTITY IN CATHOLIC HEALTH CARE: A TOPOGRAPHY

As one listens to Catholic health care—through its literature and conversations—consensus emerges around key elements of Catholic identity. These key elements constitute a "topography" of the landscape of Catholic identity. Seven central concepts and characteristics arise most often in the conversation. These are, starting with those with the highest degree of consensus:

1. Continuing the healing ministry of Jesus
2. The stories of the founding congregations

---

14. Thomas Nairn, "Not Unique, Not Distinct –Yet Catholic?: Integrity Is Key," *Health Progress* 92, no. 4 (July-August 2011): 104-6; and Carol Taylor, "The Buck Stops Here," *Health Progress* 82, no. 5 (September-October 2001): 37-40.

3. Catholic social teaching

4. Catholic health care as a ministry

5. Being in communion with the church

6. The sacramentality of Catholic health care and

7. Catholic health care and evangelization.

Beneath this topography, one can discern a "geology," the fundamental theological convictions that underlie and connect these elements, providing a multi-layered theological grounding. First, we begin with a brief discussion of each of the components of the topography.

3.2.1 THE PERSON AND WORK OF JESUS

CHA's mission statement succinctly captures a cornerstone of Catholic health care: "Catholic health care is a ministry of the Catholic Church continuing Jesus' mission of love and healing in the world today."[15] Such a claim is echoed in the mission statements of almost every Catholic health system in the U.S. and in the *Directives*. As the U.S. bishops note in the *Directives*:

> The Church has always sought to embody our Savior's
> concern for the sick….The mystery of Christ casts light
> on every facet of Catholic health care: to see Christian love
> as the animating principle of health care; to see healing
> and compassion as a continuation of Christ's mission; to
> see suffering as a participation in the redemptive power of
> Christ's passion, death, and resurrection; and to see death,
> transformed by the resurrection, as the opportunity for a
> final act of communion with Christ.[16]

---

15. CHA Mission Statement: http://www.chausa.org/Pages/Our_Work/Mission/Mission_Resources/A_Shared_Statement_of_Identity/.

16. The U. S. Conference of Catholic Bishops, *The Ethical and Religious Directives for Catholic Health Care Services,* 5ᵀᴴ edition (Washington, D.C.: USCCB Publishing, 2009). See also National Conference of Catholic Bishops, *Health and Health Care: A Pastoral Letter of the American Catholic Bishops* (Washington, D.C.: U.S. Catholic Conference,1981).

Thus, whether referring to "Gospel values," "continuing Jesus' healing ministry" or "following the example of Christ," Catholic health care firmly grounds itself in the life, mission, redemptive work and person of Jesus Christ.

At the same time, from the Gospels through mid-twentieth century America, the Christian tradition has identified the sick person with Christ. In Matthew's Gospel, Jesus commends those who visited the sick—"whatever you did for one of these least brothers of mine, you did for me" (Mt. 25:36)—and condemns those who did not. This impelled Christians from the earliest communities forward to care for the sick *as Christ.* Such a perspective shapes how one interacts with patients.

Thus, theologically, Catholic health care draws its identity from Christology.[17] Jesus has always been eminently present in the consciousness and practice of Catholic health care—in its reason for being, in the way it was practiced by the religious sisters and brothers, in the ways it has thought about patients, and more. To root Catholic health care in the person and work of Jesus requires a balanced Christology that understands Jesus both "from below" and "from above," that attends to both Jesus' human and divine natures.

---

17. A danger in Catholic health care, especially in religiously pluralistic settings, is to limit Jesus to simply his healing work in the Gospels. Jesus the compassionate healer seems uncontroversial in a pluralistic context. From the perspective of Catholic theology, however, care must be taken not to limit Jesus simply to his historical humanity. Jesus is not just an amazingly good man to be emulated but rather the Son of God who ushered in the Kingdom, the Second Person of the Trinity, the One truly present in the world in the breaking of the bread, where two or three are gathered, and in the sick, hungry, naked and imprisoned. Catholic health care continues the healing ministry of Jesus by continuing to make Christ present to the sick and their loved ones. Therefore, whenever those within Catholic health care invoke the name of "Jesus," they are at least implicitly presuming certain "Christologies." Adequate theological formation requires attention to operative background Christologies.

3.2.2. THE STORIES OF THE FOUNDERS

Alongside Jesus in the identities of Catholic health systems stand the stories of the founding religious orders—those particular women or men who founded the hospitals as well as the broader work of those who created Catholic health care as a whole. In most health systems, the stories of the founders are critical, tangible entry points to a particular Catholic ministry's narrative. When told well, they necessarily connect today's associates to the founders' experience of Christ and the ways they embodied that experience of Jesus in the world.[18]

These stories are important in three ways. First, stories are foundational to identity. We are all shaped by particular stories and narratives.[19] Often, the stories that most powerfully drive our actions do so implicitly. We adopt them from the world around us, and they shape our lives and actions without our realizing it. As such, we are always shaped by multiple stories. Operative in our own institutions are the narratives of medicine and the various professions; free market economics; American identity; cultural stories about health, illness, poverty and death; local histories; as well as the stories of our founding religious orders, the longer history of Catholic health care and the broader Catholic tradition as well. Some of these stories may overlap; often they are in conflict. Getting one's stories straight is a first step in clarifying identity.

What is more, stories in the Catholic tradition have theological significance. Sr. Juliana Casey, IHM, STD, Ph.D., a longtime leader in Catholic health care, refers to the repeated return to the founders' stories as a practice of "holy memory." As she notes:

---

18. I wish to thank Ron Mead, chief mission officer, St.Vincent Health, Indianapolis, for this and many other insights incorporated into this study.

19. Ron Hamel, "The Stories We Live by," *Health Progress* 89, no. 3 (May-June 2008): 14-5.

> Remembering is one of the most important themes in the Judeo-Christian tradition....To remember within a faith context is to do more than recall an event: It is to reenter the event, to become present to the grace and power it manifests.[20]

This sort of remembering—a remembering that makes an event present—is what Catholics call *anamnesis*. *Anamnesis* is at the heart of the Eucharist. When we "do this in remembrance" of Jesus, we reenter the event of his passion and resurrection; he becomes "really present" to those gathered to worship. Similarly, those who work in Catholic health care recall the stories of the founders anamnetically— not simply as quaint, historical artifacts, but as incarnations of grace that they re-enter, bringing that grace and power forward, embodying the founders' charisms in new contexts.

Such *anamnesis* is the work of the Holy Spirit. Equally, the charisms of religious congregations—in this case, the founders of Catholic health care—are particular conduits for the power of the Spirit to work for the good of the church and the world.[21] The 2002 Vatican document *Starting Afresh from Christ* speaks of the energy of the Spirit embodied in charisms: "Consecrated life, like all forms of Christian life, is by its nature *dynamic*....It came into being through *the creative prompting of the Spirit* who moved the founders and foundresses along the Gospel path."[22] Consonant with the powerful insight of Catholic health care, theologian Fr. Bernard Lee, SM, Th.D., ties these charisms back to what he calls "the deep stories" of the communities that arise in a particular social and historical context,

---

20. Juliana Casey, "Holy Memory, Faithful Action," *Health Progress* 81, (March-April 2000): 28-31.

21. This account of charism is drawn from Sr. Marlene Weisenbeck's article, "Understanding Charism," *Health Progress* 89, no. 6 (November-December 2008): 16-7. The points of contact between her account of charism and this overview on Catholic identity are striking. In particular, she identifies criteria by which a charism can be recognized. In addition to the Spirit's role, she includes "fidelity in witnessing to some aspect of the Trinitarian Mystery," "the evangelical intent of the founders," being conformed to Christ, ecclesial awareness, and "openness to discernment and confirmation by the Church."

22. Congregation for Institutes of Consecrated Life and Societies of Apostolic Life, *Starting Afresh from Christ,* May 19, 2002, 20.

but notes that as these "deep stories" meet new social contexts, it is the work of the Spirit to bring the essence of the charism forward in a new and fitting way. It is again a work of *anamnesis*.[23]

QUESTIONS FOR REFLECTION AND DISCUSSION

1. Catholic identity is associated with the following elements: attending to the relationships with the diocesan bishop and the sponsor(s), following the *Ethical and Religious Directives for Health Care Services*, offering strong pastoral care and mission services, offering the sacraments, providing a significant level of charity care and community benefit. What elements are considered necessary for health care organizations to maintain their Catholic identity? What other elements do you believe express your organization's Catholic identity?

2. If integrity is based on how our actions reflect who we say we are, how can leadership assure integrity of action and identity in large, multifaceted and geographically distant Catholic health care systems?

3. If we claim that our ministry is rooted in the person and the work of Jesus, and that we are committed to continue his healing ministry and to see Christ in those who are served, how might we affiliate with organizations that are not founded on the person of Jesus?

4. How might structural change, mergers and affiliations affect a Catholic health care ministry's founding narrative? How do

---

23. Charisms and the gifts of the Holy Spirit are not limited to vowed religious but are, of course, made available to all the faithful, including lay persons who work in Catholic health care. See *Lumen Gentium* § 12: "It is not only through the sacraments and the ministries of the Church that the Holy Spirit sanctifies and leads the people of God and enriches it with virtues, but, 'allotting His gifts to everyone according as He wills' (1 Cor 12:11). He distributes special graces among the faithful of every rank. By these gifts He makes them fit and ready to undertake the various tasks and offices which contribute toward the renewal and building up of the Church, according to the words of the Apostle: 'The manifestation of the Spirit is given to everyone for profit'" (Cf 1 Thess 5:12, 12-21). This affirmation of the charisms given to lay persons is critically important for developing an account of lay leadership of Catholic health care.

the "deep stories" meet new social contexts in order to bring the charism of the founders forward in a new and fitting way?

3.2.3 CATHOLIC SOCIAL PRINCIPLES

Along with continuing the work of Jesus and the founders, the principles of Catholic social thought hold primacy of place in a survey of the hallmarks of Catholic identity. Again, mission statements, working group statements and a myriad of articles on Catholic identity in Catholic health care champion the principles of the Catholic social tradition. Again and again, we hear of human dignity, care for the whole person, care for the poor and vulnerable, the common good, stewardship, solidarity, subsidiarity, participation and more.[24] The centrality of these principles is affirmed in the *Directives,* particularly Part I, as well as the National Conference of Catholic Bishops' pastoral letter on *Health and Health Care.*[25]

This body of Catholic Church teaching, which took a new form with Pope Leo XIII's encyclical *Rerum Novarum* (1891), grew in breadth and depth over the 20th century, especially as articulated in the teachings of popes and bishops as well as theologians and bishops in Latin America.[26] Although the principles themselves trace a long history in scripture and the Christian tradition, they come to be articulated in a new way in this body of teaching. Pope by pope, Catholic social thought moves forward by responding to particular, concrete issues as they arise: the debilitating effects of the industrial revolution on workers *(Rerum Novarum)*, the threat of nuclear war *(Pacem in Terris)*, the shift from colonialism to development

---

24. For just a few examples, see Ed Giganti, "Living Our Promises, Acting on Faith," *Health Progress* 82, no. 1 (January-February 2001): 32; Francis G. Morrisey, "Catholic Identity in a Challenging Environment," *Health Progress* 80, no.6 (November-December 1999): 38-42; Michael D. Place, "Catholic Identity: A Unifying Force," *Health Progress* 80, no. 2 (March-April 1999): 10, 14; Richard Haughian 2004; and Doris Gottemoeller, "Preserving Our Catholic Identity," *Health Progress* 80, no. 3 (May-June 1999): 18-21.

25. NCCB, *Health and Health Care.*

26. For more information on Catholic social teaching, including key documents, see the website of Education for Justice: https://educationforjustice.org/catholic-social-teaching-resources.

as an international model *(Populorum Progressio)*, the development of globalization and the negative impacts of neoliberal economic practices *(Sollicitudo Rei Socialis)*, the economic crisis of 2008 *(Caritas in Veritate)* and more.

This responsiveness to the signs of the times and emergent issues has made the Catholic social tradition particularly appealing to Catholic health care, which likewise has always found itself responding to changing contexts and new questions. Equally, the Catholic social tradition emerged and grew concurrent with the development of Catholic health care in the U.S., and alongside the emergence of new lay movements in the 20TH century. Lay persons and those commited to Catholic health care have thus, often, had a special affection for Catholic social thought. Its principles have come to "infuse the marrow" of Catholic health care in so many ways—in employee compensation and benefits; in the rights of employees to organize and form unions; in employee policies in general; in billing practices; and, of course, in charity care and community benefit.[27]

Yet as we will see in Part VI, the Catholic social tradition may well pose important challenges to the current structures of Catholic health care. We will return to the principles in our discussion of for-profit health care, outlining many of them in greater detail.

3.2.4 CATHOLIC HEALTH CARE AS A MINISTRY

Catholic health care strongly affirms that it is a "ministry." Yet the term "ministry" as applied to the work of lay persons in the world is a very recent theological development. Although new lay initiatives such as Catholic Action energized the first half of the 20TH century, prior to Vatican II, "there was no official teaching about the place of

---

27. Sr. Doris Gottemoeller deserves the credit for this wonderful metaphor for the principles and Catholic health care.

28. Charles E. Bouchard, "Health Care as 'Ministry': Common Usage, Confused Theology," *Health Progress* 89, no. 3 (May-June 2008): 26; and Zeni Fox, "Making All Things New: Catholic Health Care, the Laity, and the Church," *Health Progress* 95, no. 5 (September-October 2011): 13.

the lay faithful in the life of the church."[28] The first major theological treatise on the laity was that by Fr. Yves Congar, OP, *Lay People and the Church* (1953). It is only after Vatican II that the term "ministry" comes to be applied to lay people. Even in *Lumen Gentium*—the Dogmatic Constitution on the Church—the term "ministry" remains reserved for priests; the work of the laity in the world continues to be referred to as an "apostolate." But with *Lumen Gentium,* the sacramental basis of Christian work in the world shifts from ordination to Baptism, even for priests and consecrated religious.[29] This baptismal grounding of what is eventually subsumed under the term ministry is reaffirmed in the United States Conference of Catholic Bishops' 2005 document on lay ministry entitled *Co-Workers in the Vineyard of the Lord* in which "the centrality of Baptism is stressed because it makes us members of the Body of Christ, initiates us to the Christian community, and calls us to a holiness of life....The role of the laity in ministry is grounded in Baptism."[30] To be rooted in Baptism reflects the Catholic conviction that the ministry of lay persons is, by definition, ecclesial.

Dominican ethicist Fr. Charles E. Bouchard, STD, draws on the work of theologian Fr. Thomas O'Meara, OP, Ph.D., who defines lay ecclesial ministry as "the public activity of a baptized follower of Jesus Christ, flowing from the Spirit's charism and an individual personality on behalf of a Christian community to proclaim, serve and realize the Kingdom of God."[31] In addition, lay ministers, at least to some extent, "act officially on behalf of the church; and have, to varying degrees, an ecclesial status."[32]

However, while lay initiatives have blossomed since Vatican II, this notion of lay ministry is still in an early stage of development. Some official church documents still seem very mixed about the validity

---

29. Fox, 2011, 13; and Bouchard, 2008, 27. See *Lumen Gentium*, §33.

30. Fox, 2011, 14.

31. Bouchard, 2008, 26.

32. Bouchard.

of lay ecclesial ministry, describing it more as a stop-gap remedy until there are enough priests rather than a proper expression of baptismal dignity.[33] In both theory and practice, the balance and mutuality of official and lay authority has not yet fully emerged.[34]

If the notion of lay ministry is relatively new, the question of whether an *institution* can be considered a ministry is even newer. Although institutions of service—including Catholic hospitals—have been run by Catholics for centuries, Fr. Bouchard maintains that "until recently these institutions were usually not considered 'ministries' in the proper sense."[35] Usually, as activities of religious institutes, they too were considered apostolates and were theologized under the umbrella of religious life. This connection to religious congregations provided an ecclesial identity for the work of Catholic health care. Moreover, while the histories of Catholic health care often highlight the role of individual women and men religious, it has been the congregations that have allowed the founders to sustain and continue the ministry over time—even centuries.

These two areas—lay ecclesial ministry and the works of religious institutes—are the two main theological resources currently available for developing a theology of Catholic health care as a ministry. Neither, however, provides an exact fit with the current realities of Catholic health care. As is widely recognized, one of the tensions within Catholic health care concerns the transitioning of the work of the ministry from consecrated religious to lay persons, a transition for which there are few models outside of health care and as yet no theology. The multitude of formation programs within Catholic health systems that have been developed over the past two decades have emerged out of an attempt to address this new development.

33. Bouchard.

34. Fox, 2011, 13.

35. Bouchard, 2008, 27.

Similarly, the "ecclesial" nature of Catholic health care systems differs from that of parishes, the context presumed by most theological reflection on lay ministry. Unlike parishes, religious communities, and even many other Catholic ministries, health care institutions are religiously pluralistic—in staff, in leadership, in clientele. Many who work in Catholic health care are not baptized—some are deeply committed to the mission, some are indifferent (as are some Catholics). Many within health care *do* understand their work as a ministry, yet they have no official ecclesial standing.

Nevertheless, the theology of lay ecclesial ministry and the theology of the apostolates of religious congregations stand as necessary theological starting points for developing an account of Catholic health care institutions as ministries. Are a critical mass of the sponsor members baptized? Are they commissioned, perhaps, as sponsor members in a liturgical ceremony, receiving an ecclesial status and perhaps formally adopting the charisms of the systems' founders? Does the organization encourage associates and leaders within the organization to understand their work as part of a public activity flowing from the Spirit's charism on behalf of the Catholic Church to realize the Kingdom of God? What does it mean to do this work "on behalf of the Catholic Church"? These questions require us to address our next characteristic: what it means for Catholic health care to be "in communion with the church."

QUESTIONS FOR REFLECTION AND DISCUSSION

1. Which principles of the Catholic social tradition might appeal to new partners whose foundation is in business principles, capitalism and secularism?

2. Which principles of the Catholic social tradition might be challenging to the workings of a for-profit organization?

3. While over the past two decades leaders in Catholic health care have become familiar with the concept of "lay ministry" through

formation programs, how might the sense of lay ministry be
challenged when a Catholic health care ministry is affiliated with
an other-than-Catholic entity?

3.2.5 IN COMMUNION WITH THE CHURCH

To date, there has been a consensus that to be a Catholic health
care institution, as a ministry of the church,[36] is necessarily to be in
communion with the church. Given the evolving notion of ministry
outlined above and the developments in Catholic ecclesiology (the
theology of the church) since Vatican II, however, what exactly it
means to be "in communion with the church" has become less clear.

Catholic ecclesiology is one of union and communion. The church, as
the Body of Christ, has "many parts" but they all comprise one body.
No part of the body can exist on its own as "church" without union
and communion; all parts are equally essential. The ecclesiology of
Vatican II is referred to as "communion ecclesiology." Outlined in
Lumen Gentium particularly, this full, complex vision of the church
was meant to amend a more juridical, institutional understanding
that saw the church as the *societas perfectas* and had restricted its focus
to the magisterium.[37] Communion ecclesiology grounds the church
in a sacramental point of departure. Constituted by the baptism
of individuals into the Body of Christ, the church is created anew
each time the Eucharist is celebrated. This sacramental ecclesiology
is captured in the participatory image of the "People of God," "with
its structures of participation based on the common priesthood of
the faithful and on the charisms the Holy Spirit stirs up so that the
Church can accomplish her universal mission."[38]

---

36. For just a few examples, see Giganti 2001; Morrisey 1999; Place 1999; Haughian 2004; Casey 2000; and Gottemoeller 1999.

37. Bishop Mark Ouellet, "The Ecclesiology of Communion, 50 Years after the Opening of Vatican Council II." Available at: http://www.catholicculture.org/culture/library/view.cfm?recnum=9968.

38. Ouellet.

39. I would like to thank Sr. Jean de Blois for this important insight.

Thus, in many ways, the traditional phrase "in communion with the church" is no longer quite accurate. It would be more accurate to speak of being "in communion as church." To be *church* is to be in communion; to be a ministry of the church is to be in communion *as* church.[39]

To date, most accounts of the relationship between Catholic health care and the church do not reflect this fuller ecclesiology. Most often, those who address this relationship turn to canon law, citing the four canonical criteria for an institution to be recognized as Catholic,[40] or highlight the role of sponsorship.

Meeting the four canonical criteria permits an institution to be recognized as a Catholic organization. Canonist Fr. Francis G. Morrisey, OMI, JCD, Ph.D., reminds us of an important distinction within canon law between "Catholic works" (which are "undertaken 'in the name of the Church'" (canon 116)) and "works of Catholics," which are simply activities undertaken by Catholics and might have an ecclesial relationship or might be totally secular in their nature.[41] The Society of St. Vincent DePaul and the Knights of Columbus are lay organizations with strong Catholic identities but are not canonically recognized as Catholic. They are "works of Catholics." Canonically, Catholic works, on the other hand, must meet six conditions, in addition to the criteria mentioned above: the work must have a spiritual purpose; it must answer a genuine need; the organization must have sufficient means to carry it out; with an eye to perpetuity; guided by stewardship; and quality.[42]

---

40. These four criteria are: be guided by church authorities, be canonically established, be bound by canon law, and be subject to visitation by the diocesan bishop. See Francis G. Morrisey, "What Does Canon Law Say about the Quality of Sponsored Works?" *Health Progress* 88, no. 3 (March-April 2007): 10-11. See also Daniel Edward Pilarczyk, "Strong Catholic Identity Key to Effective Health Care Apostolate," *Hospital Progress* 61, no. 11 (November1980): 46-7.

41. Morrisey, 2007. This notion of "works of Catholics" is an underdeveloped concept in canon law and Catholic theology. It is related to the ongoing tensions within 20th and 21st century Catholicism regarding the relationships between lay initiatives and diocesan bishops. For more on this distinction, as well as various ways that health care and other organizations are negotiating these questions of ecclesial relationality, see Morrisey, "Canon Law and the Ongoing Sponsorship of Apostolic Works," presented to the CHA Collaborative Sponsor Formation Program, March 2013.

Historically, Catholic health care has considered itself a Catholic work, an extension of the work of the founding religious congregations or dioceses. The contemporary literature continues this assumption, referring to it variously as "an apostolic work,"[43] "an apostolic activity,"[44] "an extension of Christ's work and the ministry of the church,"[45] or an "instrument of God's work and healing ministry."[46]

In the 1970s, changes in both health care and religious life required new ways of structuring the continuity between Catholic health care institutions and their founding religious congregations. The new role of sponsors and public juridic persons, both developed in the 1980s, are canonical innovations designed to maintain an official connection between religious institutes, their ministries and the church. As defined in CHA's report, *Toward a Theology of Catholic Health Care Sponsorship,* sponsorship of a health care ministry is:

> a formal relationship between an authorized Catholic organization and a legally formed system, hospital, clinic, nursing home (or other institution) entered into for the sake of promoting and sustaining Christ's healing ministry to people in need.[47]

---

42. Paralleling the history of lay ministry, canonical limitations on the right to use the name "Catholic" appear to be relatively recent developments, introduced with the 1983 revision of the Code of Canon Law [See canons 216, 300, 803, and 808 as developments of AA 24] code. See Elissa Rinere, "Catholic Identity and the Use of the Name 'Catholic,' *Jurist* 62 , no.1 (2002): 131-58. As both Rinere and Morrisey observe, in spite of these canons, a simple internet search unearths "thousands of schools, associations of the faithful, or other organizations, all espousing Catholic values and identity, and none indicating whether or not they have received the required consent to use the name 'Catholic'" (Rinere, 158; see also Morrisey 2013).

43. Morrisey, 1999.

44. Morrisey, 2007.

45. Gottemoeller, 1999.

46. Place, 1999.

47. Catholic Health Association, *Toward a Theology of Catholic Health Care Sponsorship* (St. Louis: Catholic Health Association, 2005).

Originally, sponsors tended to be members of religious institutes, but as sponsorship models have continued to evolve, lay groups have increasingly been invited to become sponsors.

Sponsorship, therefore, has served as an important model of communion *as* church. As the CHA report notes, sponsorship begins to address the inexact fit between Catholic health care, ecclesial lay ministry and theologies of religious apostolates:

> Although the Church is certainly present among the people of God who work in health care—in their values and motivation and style of giving care—their contribution still remains the work of individuals unless it is officially authorized by the Church. Once the work is authorized, however, the same individuals act not only as baptized Christians following Christ, but as part of an institution with a mandate to minister *in the Church's name*.[48]

The practice of sponsorship begins to move Catholic health care toward a more complete understanding of theology of the church—one that begins to theologize institutions as ministries and to incorporate the work of laity into a fuller vision of the shared work of lay, vowed religious and diocesan bishops.

It also developed in part to address unclarity about the relationship between Catholic health systems and diocesan bishops, particularly in light of the variability of episcopal interpretation of moral norms across dioceses. Traditionally, Catholic health care has recognized that to claim to be a "Catholic" ministry has required validation of that identity by a diocesan bishop as an expression of communion and union.[49] Catholic ecclesiology locates responsibility for the unity

---

48. CHA, *Toward a Theology of Catholic Health Care Sponsorship*.

49. Sr. Doris Gottemoeller helpfully outlines three requirements for Catholic identity: assertion, validation and integration. "For Profit and Catholic? How Would the Ministry Fare?" *Health Progress 93*, no 4 (July-August 2012): 31-5.

of the local church and the exercise of all ministry within it with
the diocesan bishop. Yet different bishops draw on different images
of the church, on, that is, different aspects of Catholic ecclesiology,
as they envisage the relationship between the diocesan bishop and
local health care institutions.[50] Different images, all warranted by
Vatican II, provide different nuances for the role of the laity and their
relationship with the diocesan bishop. Equally, lay persons and many
in Catholic health care draw on this same variety of ecclesiologies.
However, as Cardinal Avery Dulles, SJ, STD, notes in his classic book
Models of the Church "a balanced theology of the Church must find a
way of incorporating the major affirmations" of the variety of images
and models validated by Vatican II. To overemphasize any one aspect
of the church to the exclusion of the others will lead to distortions,
contributing to unfortunate divisions and dissension within the
church.[51] As with Christology, for health care to identify as Catholic
requires a balanced ecclesiology.

Thus, the question of how the relationship between the diocesan
bishop and Catholic health care ought best be structured remains to
be more clearly defined. Bishops played a key role in the founding
of Catholic hospitals in the early history of Catholic health care in
the U.S. Throughout the 19TH and 20TH centuries, they served on the
boards of hospitals. Yet today, the concrete manner of relationship
is not clear. Many who are involved in Catholic ministries would
welcome greater involvement in their work on the part of the
diocesan bishop. The *Directives* and the bishops' pastoral letter
on *Health and Health Care* provide guidance for clarifying and
strengthening these relationships. What is more, beyond the office of

50. When speaking of the relationship between bishops and Catholic health care, bishops invoke a variety of images: the Body of Christ, pilgrim people, community of disciples, hierarchical institution or communion ecclesiology. See, for example: Donald Wuerl, "Catholic Health Ministry in Transition," *Health Progress* 80, no. 3 (May-June 1999): 15; William Skylstad, "Catholic Health Care's Identity and Integrity," *Origins* 36, no. 6 (2006): 85-93; Bernardin 1991; Gerald Kicanas, "Creating an Ecclesial Culture of Dialogue within Catholic Healthcare," *Origins* 41, no. 39 (February 9, 2012): 570-5; Thomas H. Vowell, "Preserving Catholic Identity in Mergers," *Health Progress* 73, no. 3 (1992): 28-33; Pilarczyk, 1980; and Joseph M. Sullivan, "Ministering Together," *Health Progress* 83, no. 4 (July-August 2002): 44. Here Bishop Sullivan develops implications of Pope John Paul's *Novo Millennio Inuente* for health care.

51. Avery Dulles, *Models of the Church* (New York: Image Books, 1991), p. 2.

bishop, how else might communion with the church be constituted? Are there other ways that Catholic identity might be validated? Would alternative modes of validation compromise the fundamental theological commitment to union and communion? In what ways are Catholic hospitals in relationship with local parishes? Are Catholic health systems "in communion" with each other or fundamentally competitive? Clearly, questions abound, calling for further theological work in this area.

3.2.6. THE SACRAMENTALITY OF CATHOLIC HEALTH CARE

Central to Catholic theology, tradition, thought, practice and life is sacramentality. Catholic identity in health care must attend to its relationship to sacraments and sacramentality.[52]

As noted earlier, the ministry of Catholic health care is grounded in Christology—in the person and work of Christ. Prior to his healing acts attested in the Gospels, Jesus' mission of love and healing begins with the Incarnation. Jesus is God incarnate, Word made flesh, who in his person reveals the transcendent God as love and compassion. Jesus, as theologian Fr. Edward Schillebeeckx, OP, STD, would say, is the sacrament of God: "Jesus is the perceptible sign of God's love, the embodiment of God's compassionate grace."[53]

For the Catholic theological tradition, Jesus' sacramental presence is continued in the church—the Body of Christ. Through the Spirit, Jesus commissions the church to be the visible sign, the sacrament, of God's salvation. This claim that the church is a sacrament of Christ opens *Lumen Gentium:* "the Church is in Christ like a sacrament or

---

52. Bouchard, 1999; Clarke E. Cochran, "Renewing the Sacramental," *Health Progress* 84, no. 6 (November-December 2003): 12-15; The Catholic Bishops of New Jersey, "The Rationale of Catholic Health Care," *Origins* 25, no. 27 (1995).

53. Cochran, 2003, 12; see also Cochran, "Institutional Identity: Sacramental Potential: Catholic Healthcare at Century's End," *Christian Bioethics* 5, no. 1 (1999): 34.

54. *Lumen Gentium,* §1; and Cochran, 2003, 12.

as a sign and instrument both of a very closely knit union with God and of the unity of the whole human race."[54] Therefore, the church, in all its actions—its words, its service to the poor, its ministries, its liturgies, and more—is charged to embody Christ, to make Christ visible to the world, and in so doing to be a perceptible sign of God's love and compassionate grace for the world.

Central to sacramentality is the liturgy. Daily, the sacraments renew the church. They ground the ministerial vocations of the faithful, seeking to transform us into the likeness of Christ so we can bear that likeness into the world. Both Catholic persons and Catholic institutions—specifically Catholic health care—have a vocation to embody this incarnational and participatory sacramentality. Catholics hold that the sacraments truly make Christ present. Therefore, Catholic persons and institutions are called to incarnate, embody, truly make Christ present in the world, enabled by the grace that comes through their participation in the sacramental life of the church.

To continue Jesus' mission of healing and love, therefore, is to be sacramental—to be perceptible signs of God's love, embodiments of God's compassionate grace, to signify and make real the presence of God's grace.[55] From the start, Catholic health care incorporated the sacraments into their institutional lives as an essential part of pastoral care. Thus, they provided Eucharist, chapel facilities and the sacraments of reconciliation, anointing, baptism, and even confirmation and matrimony where needed as an integral part of Catholic health care and healing. Thus, Catholic hospitals, staff and patients have always been eminently and sacramentally connected to the broader church.

Beyond the seven sacraments, however, sacramentality is incarnated in and through ordinary moments, things, and actions in the day-to-day work of hospitals and clinics. Like bread and water in the

55. Cochran, 2003, 12.

sacraments, sacramentality is mediated through ordinary aspects and actions in health care. Hospital food, wiping the drool from the chin of an Alzheimer's patient, covering a naked patient, and the multitude of actions and encounters in day-to-day care—all of these can be sacramental moments, can become "occasions of grace."[56] Thus, Catholic health care ministry is sacramental in that it effects what it symbolizes: the healing ministry of Christ.

3.2.7 CATHOLIC HEALTH CARE AND WITNESSING TO THE FAITH

Of late, a connection is made more frequently between Catholic health care and evangelization. In 2012, Bishop Ronald Gainer, JCL, of Lexington, Ky., stated at a conference entitled "Catholic Health Care: The Church's Work of Evangelization," that "the Church exists to evangelize and Catholic health care is fundamentally an expression of the Church's work of evangelization."[57] In November 2012, the Vatican Pontifical Council for Health Care Ministry sponsored a conference entitled, "The Hospital, Setting for Evangelization: A Human and Spiritual Mission."[58]

This linking of health care and evangelization makes many uncomfortable. Patients are vulnerable, at a power disadvantage relative to health care staff, and come to health care facilities for treatment of their bodies, not to be proselytized. If evangelization is equated with proselytization, this concern would be on-target. Yet the Catholic tradition clearly rejects this equation. If this is the case, what would "evangelization" mean in the health care context?

---

56. Charles E. Bouchard, "Catholic Healthcare and the Common Good," *Health Progress* 80, no. 3 (May-June 1999): 39.

57. Catholic Conference of Kentucky, "Catholic Health Care and the Church's Work of Evangelization," http://ccky.org/2012/10/catholic-health-care-the-churchs-work-of-evangelization/.

58. Catholic News Service, "Health Is Universal Good To Be Defended, not Commoditized, Says Pope," November 19, 2012. http://www.catholicnews.com/data/stories/cns/1204884.htm.

The new evangelization was a key theme of Vatican II. *Lumen Gentium* proclaims that all members of the church, and all its ministries and institutions, share in this mission: "...the whole Church is missionary, and the work of evangelization is a basic duty of the People of God"[83].[59] This theme is vibrantly continued by Popes Paul VI, John Paul II, and Benedict.[60]

An important question is whether this emphasis on evangelization comes from within or outside of Catholic health care. Historians make clear that throughout its history, evangelization was central to Catholic health care in the U.S. Christopher Kaufman's important book *Ministry and Meaning* details the complex and nuanced ways in which nursing sisters negotiated this question. Certainly, a hallmark of Catholic health care throughout its history was its unusual openness to persons of all or no faiths. Some Catholic hospitals specifically prohibited clergy of any denomination (including Catholic priests) from proselytizing the patients, holding (in the 1850s) that "the rights of conscience must be held paramount to all others.'"[61] Yet at the same time, written guidebooks for nursing sisters over this 150-year history speak of their responsibility to pray for deathbed conversions, often through stealth means such as hiding holy medals under patients' pillows. In personal letters, many sisters glowingly testify about Catholics who, due to the gracious care they received, return to the church or patients who convert—*not* because they were proselytized but due to the silent witness and prayers of the nursing sisters.[62]

---

59. Frans Jozef van Beeck, *Catholic Identity after Vatican II: Three Types of Faith in the One Church*, Campion book (Chicago: Loyola University Press, 1985).

60. On the tenth anniversary of Vatican II, Pope Paul convoked the Synod on Evangelization in the Modern World, and issued the apostolic exhortation, *Evangelii Nuntiandi*, which asserts in a new way the centrality of evangelization to the church. Pope John Paul, who helped draft *Evangelii Nuntiandi*, continued this theme throughout his own pontificate. From *Christifideles Laici* (1988) and *Redemptor Missio* (1990) through *Novo Millennio Ineunte* (2001), he reiterates and develops this theme. For more on Pope John Paul's work on evangelization see Richard Rymarz, "John Paul II and the 'New Evangelization': Origins and Meaning," *Australian eJournal of Theology* 15 (no. 1) 2010. Available at: http://aejt.com.au/__data/assets/pdf_file/0009/225396/Rymarcz_evangelization_GH.pdf.

61. Kauffman, 76.

As late as 1940, the president of the Catholic Hospital Association, Fr. Alphonse Schwitalla, SJ, Ph.D., confidently asserts, in an outline of the fundamentals of Catholic identity: "the third area of identity is the Catholic hospital's understanding that 'all human activity must be considered as means to the supernatural, and, namely the salvation of souls, then surely the functions of the hospital must be so considered.'"[63] Thus, as historian Jay P. Dolan, Ph.D., notes, "the opportunity to save souls was a primary reason so many young women became nursing sisters."[64] In adopting this position, those in Catholic health care were continuing a tradition that stretched back at least to monastic medicine, if not the early church.

Thus, the question seems not so much to be about the whether Catholic health care should witness to the faith; rather, it seems to be a matter of how. Contemporary voices from within Catholic health care agree that such witness is an important dimension of the ministry. Fr. Bouchard maintains that, rooted in the healing ministry of Jesus, the purpose of Catholic health care is "first of all to proclaim the Gospel on behalf of the church."[65] In other words, to understand Catholic health care as a ministry means that one of its functions is to witness to the Gospel in the world, to help realize the Kingdom of God by cooperating with grace in its work for the common good.[66] Cochran sees this witness rooted in the thick sense of sacramentality outlined in the previous section. Speaking of the public face of Catholic sacramentality, he argues:

> Another way of putting this is in terms of witness…no
> Catholic institution is justified unless it represents or reflects

---

62. Shortly after the turn of the 20TH century, Mother Francis Xavier Cabrini reports to the Sacred Congregation for the Propagation of the Faith on the work of Columbus Hospital in New York: "The principal goal of the hospital is to assure that the poor who have come to the end of their lives and resources find not only alleviation for their corporal misery, but principally help for their souls. Experience has shown that the majority of these people have been far away from the Church for many years. Others, even though adults, have not been baptized, nor have they received their First Holy Communion. There are also many who were not married in church. It is a consolation to see that many patients leave the hospital having been reconciled with God as well as having been helped physically" (Kauffman, 147).

63. Kauffman, 224.

64. Jay P. Dolan, "The Church and America," *Health Progress* 83, no. 4 (July-August 2002): 39.

66. Bouchard, 29.

the Kingdom of God; that is, institutions are to be "icons" of Christ…The political, policy, and institutional task of the Church is to represent a different vision of the way the world truly is and, in aspiration, can be, a vision through the lens of the crucified and risen Lord.[67]

Ministries of the church share in this task to present a different vision of the way the world is and a different way of implementing a good, such as health care, amidst the tensions of the world. By making the healing presence of God real and effective through everyday encounters, countless associates in Catholic health care quietly yet powerfully lead people to God. This form of witness, rather than proselytization, is true evangelization.

QUESTIONS FOR REFLECTION AND DISCUSSION

1. Considering the differences between "Catholic works" and "works of Catholics," what are the defining characteristics of each? Which establish more robust criteria?

2. When a ministry is authorized as a work of the church it is mandated to minister in the church's name. What responsibilities does that place upon the sponsor of the ministry? What responsibilities does it place on those in governance?

3. Theologically speaking, a Catholic health ministry may be called a sacrament of God, a perceptible sign and embodiment of God's grace. Cite some ways that sacramentality is mediated through the daily actions and ordinary aspects of the work of the ministry.

4. The Catholic tradition rejects the notion that evangelization is the same as proselytization. What is the difference, and how can a Catholic health ministry evangelize without proselytizing?

---

67. Cochran, 1999, 34.

3.3 THEOLOGICAL FOUNDATIONS OF CATHOLIC IDENTITY

Thus, as one surveys the landscape of Catholic health care, these aforementioned seven characteristics emerge as constants with regard to Catholic identity. Yet what underlies them? How are they connected to each other? What, in other words, are the *theological foundations* that undergird this landscape, giving it solidity and depth that allow it to respond dynamically yet with integrity to new developments on the surface?

To answer this question, let us step back from the topography to examine the "geology." In doing so, the two-dimensional "map" begins to take on a three-dimensional depth. We can begin to see layers. We can begin to see that not all the surface characteristics are equal, but that some are rooted in others. We can also begin to discern the center of this foundation, the core theological reality, that informs all the other characteristics.

Using the above metaphor, imagine Catholic identity as a sphere with concentric layers. At the outermost level—the level of visible behaviors—we find the stories of the founders of Catholic health care and the principles of Catholic social thought. These are the tangible manifestations—the mountain ranges, if you will—of the topography of Catholic identity. Immediately undergirding these are the theological concepts of ministry and evangelization, the grounding for both Catholic social thought and the work of religious communities. Undergirding ministry and evangelization, we find the fundamental doctrines of sacramentality and ecclesiology, both of which are necessarily rooted in Christology—the person and work of Christ. And at the center of it all, at the heart of Catholic identity in Catholic health care, is charity or *caritas*—the fundamental theological reality: that God is love, that God so loved the world. *Caritas*—love or charity—shares the same root as the word *grace* (cháris). God's essence—revealed in the Trinity, in every action of God toward humanity and the world—is *caritas* in communion.

A graphic representation of the interrelationships between these theological concepts might be sketched as follows:

Grounding of Catholic Identity

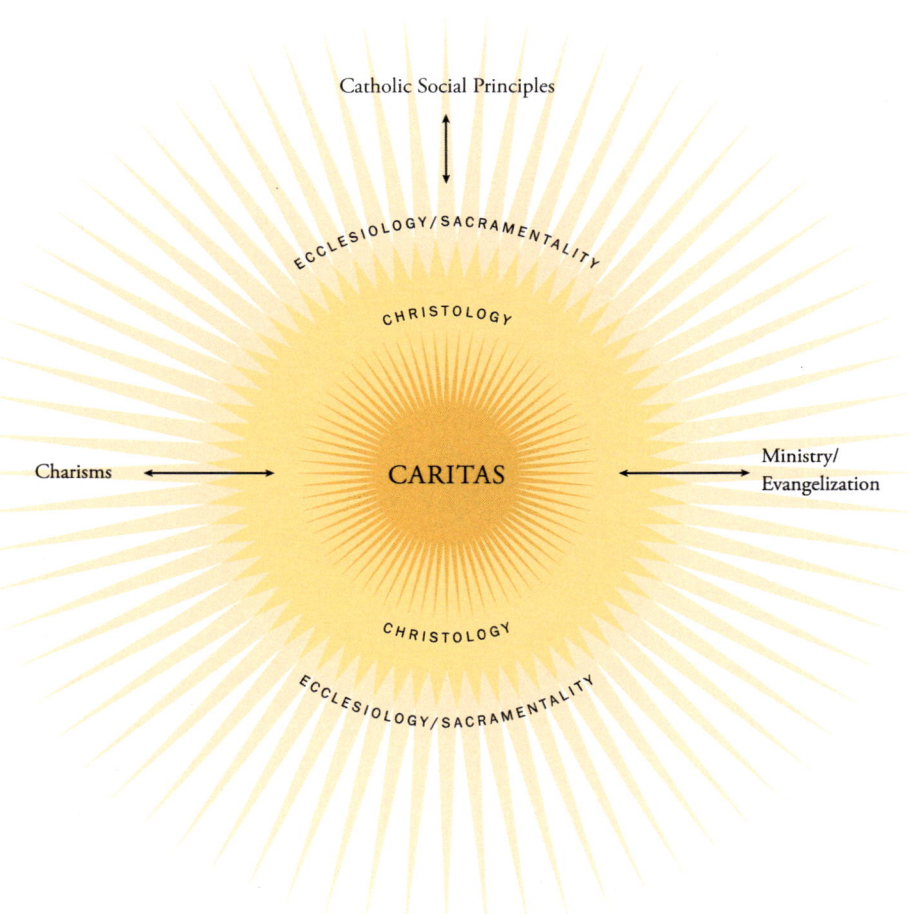

This image captures two important points. The first is that any theological foundation for Catholic identity in Catholic health care is—and must be—multi-faceted. No one theological doctrine or conviction stands on its own; they cannot be separated from each other. Second, there is a dynamic relationship between the elements of this multi-faceted foundation. *Caritas* shapes our understanding of Jesus, the church, Catholic social thought and more. The principles of Catholic social thought or of Spirit-given charisms should inform our understanding of church. All the components can deepen our understanding of God's love and work in the world. And so forth.

Caritas as the foundational theological reality of Catholic health care is attested best in Bishop William Skylstad's powerful address to the Catholic Health Assembly in 2006 entitled "Catholic Health Care's Identity and Integrity."[68] There, Bishop Skylstad, then bishop of Spokane, Wash., draws heavily on Pope Benedict's first encyclical *Deus Caritas Est*, God Is Love (2005). Bishop Skylstad did not have available to him Pope Benedict's most recent encyclical, *Caritas in Veritate*, Charity in Truth (2009), which provides an even more extensive vision of the work of *caritas* in the world.

Thus, at the heart of Catholic health care lies *caritas*, God's gracious love made present in the world through the work of caregivers, associates and senior leadership. *Caritas* in communion as the fundamental theological reality should inform, infuse and transform every aspect of Catholic health care, every action, every structure, every practice. Too often, when we speak of "charity" in relationship to Catholic health care, it becomes monetized—referring primarily to "charity care" or "uncompensated care." Or we equate it with "caring for the poor." While these are certainly components of *caritas*, they are only one part. The following snapshots indicate the multiple ways that the theological notion of *caritas* goes beyond simply "charity care," as well as the way in which it constantly moves toward the creation of communion.

---

68. William Skylstad, "Catholic Health Care's Identity and Integrity," *Origins* 36, no. 6 (June 22, 2006): 85-93.

+ **Charity as God's Essence:** In both *Deus Caritas Est* and *Caritas in Veritate*, Pope Benedict makes clear that the theological foundation of all reality, of Christianity, of the Catholic tradition—and by extrapolation the work of Catholic health care—is *charity* understood as God's essence and God's essential and actual way of being and interacting with the world. God's act of creation in Genesis, God's ongoing sustaining of creation, God's every interaction with creation and humanity is, in its essence, charity enacted in and creating communion. It is gift. It is self-gift. It is love. It is creative, redemptive, transformative, reconciling. It is the essence of the Trinity. As Pope Benedict elaborates: "Charity is love received and given. It is 'grace' (*cháris*). Its source is the wellspring of the Father's love for the Son, in the Holy Spirit. Love comes down to us from the Son. It is creative love, through which we have our being; it is redemptive love, through which we are recreated. Love is revealed and made present by Christ (cf. Jn 13:1) and 'poured into our hearts through the Holy Spirit' (Rom 5:5). As the objects of God's love, men and women become subjects of charity, they are called to make themselves instruments of grace, so as to pour forth God's charity and to weave networks of charity" (*Caritas in Veritate*, §5).

+ **Charity as the Essence of the Person and Work of Christ:** As the Second Person of the Trinity, the being and work of Christ Jesus can be none other than, in essence, charity as well. Through the Incarnation, his work and the Passion, Jesus reveals *caritas* to be self-gift, and, more specifically, self-emptying (Phil. 2:5). Through *caritas*, Jesus enters into communion with humanity, taking on human nature. The gospels witness his constant creation of communion—with the disciples, with those on the margins, even with those who persecute him. Through Jesus, communion with God—redemption—is made possible.

+ **Charity as the Essence of the Sacraments:** Necessary for becoming agents of *caritas* are ongoing encounters with the God who loves us.

Echoing many who reflect on Catholic health care, Pope Benedict emphasizes the need for personal spiritual formation rooted in the sacraments. "Consequently, in addition to their necessary professional training, these charity workers need a 'formation of the heart': They need to be led to that encounter with God in Christ which awakens their love and opens their spirits to others…they must be persons moved by Christ's love, persons whose hearts Christ has conquered with his love, awakening within them a love of neighbor" (*Deus Caritas Est*, §31, 33). The place we encounter this God who loves in this creative, redemptive, kenotic way is the communion of Eucharist and prayer (*Deus Caritas Est*, §13). This communion empowers us to extend communion to patients and co-workers.

+ **Charity as the Essence of the Church:** Pope Benedict's sacramental theology entails a vision of the church. The Eucharist, he maintains (in good company with many sacramental theologians), connects all who participate in the celebration, whether they are physically present to each other or not: "…this sacramental 'mysticism' is social in character, for in sacramental communion, I become one with the Lord, like all the other communicants. As Saint Paul says, 'Because there is one bread, we who are many are one body, for we all partake of the one bread' (1 Cor 10:17). Union with Christ is also union with all those to whom he gives himself. I cannot possess Christ just for myself; I can belong to him only in union with all those who have become, or who will become, his own. Communion draws me out of myself towards him, and thus also towards unity with all Christians. We become 'one body,' completely joined in a single existence" (*Deus Caritas Est*, §14).

+ **Charity as the Essence of Ministry:** This interweaving of Christology, sacraments and church overflows into the world via the laity: "Faith, worship and ethos are interwoven as a single reality which takes shape in our encounter with God's agape. Here the usual [distinction] between worship and ethics simply falls apart. Worship itself, Eucharistic communion, includes the reality both of being loved and of loving others in turn. *A Eucharist which does not pass over into the concrete practice of love is intrinsically fragmented"* (*Deus Caritas Est*, §14, emphasis added). Those who work in Catholic health care continue the work of Jesus, enabled by the Spirit, because we have first been objects of *caritas*—we have first received God's love and grace. Thus, we can become "instruments of grace," we can "weave networks of charity"—in every single action we take, not just in caring for the poor or providing uncompensated care.

+ **Charity as the Essence of Witness:** Bishop Skylstad makes clear that Pope Benedict warns against using charity as a means of proselytization (*Deus Caritas Est*, §31). Rather, the heart of evangelization is loving presence, sometimes silent: "A Christian knows when it is time to speak of God and when it is better to say nothing and to let love alone speak. He knows that ... God's presence is felt at the very time when the only thing we do is to love....It is the responsibility of the Church's charitable organizations to reinforce this awareness in their members, so that by their activity — as well as their words, their silence, their example — they may be credible witnesses to Christ" (*Deus Caritas Est*, §31).

+ **Charity as the Essence of Catholic Social Principles:** For St. Thomas Aquinas, "charity is the form of the virtues"—it transforms mere human or natural virtues into theological practices, so that in the end, for Thomas, the Christian moral life is really a life of charity. Pope Benedict sees a similar dynamic at work with the social principles: "Charity is at the heart of the Church's social doctrine. Every responsibility and every commitment spelled out by that doctrine is derived from charity which, according to the teaching of Jesus, is the synthesis of the entire Law (cf. Mt 22:36- 40). It gives real substance to the personal relationship with God and with neighbor; it is the principle not only of micro-relationships (with friends, with family members or within small groups) but also of macro-relationships (social, economic and political ones)" (*Caritas in Veritate*, §2).[69]

+ **Charity and the Founders' Stories:** The stories of the amazing women and men who responded to human need, to epidemics, wars, urban poverty, frontier isolation and more are primarily stories of charity, of caring for the poor. Pope Benedict asserts again and again in *Deus Caritas Est* and *Caritas in Veritate* that this exercise of charity—"love for widows, orphans, prisoners, the sick and needy of every kind"—has from its very beginnings, been one of the church's essential activities or responsibilities, along with administering the sacraments and proclaiming the Gospel: "The Church cannot neglect the service of charity anymore than she can neglect the sacraments and the word... These duties presuppose each other and are inseparable" (*Deus Caritas Est*, §22, 25). "For the Church, charity is not a kind of welfare activity which could equally well be left to others, but is a part of her nature, an indispensable expression of her very being" (*Deus Caritas Est*, §25). The practical charity embodied by the founders and Catholic health care institutions today is indispensable to the very being of the church, inseparable from its other ecclesial responsibilities. Moreover, the term "charity" describes not only the outreach of the founders to the poor they encountered; it describes also the shape of their caring—as it was premised on their own gift of self. Living in solidarity with those they cared for, taking little or no money, their entire lives were acts of charity.

We find, then, a multi-layered theological foundation for Catholic identity in Catholic health care. Catholic health care as a concrete practice of love takes the shape of communion (ministry, evangelization and Catholic social thought captured in the Spirit-led

---

69. Pope Benedict traces this insight back to Pope Paul in *Populorum Progressio*, noting that "*In the notion of development, understood in human and Christian terms, he [Paul VI] identified the heart of the Christian social message*, and he proposed Christian charity as the principal force at the service of development" (*Caritas in Veritate*, §13, emphasis in original).

charisms of the founders of our systems) grounded in a sacramentality which is intertwined with ecclesiology, both of which are rooted in Christology, the summit and fullness of the revelation of God's *caritas* in world.[70]

Which emerging models of health care delivery can best capture such an identity? There is certainly more than one answer. And particular models may well diminish a system's ability to live these commitments. For most of the past 30 years, one tool for assessing the fit between system structure and Catholic identity has been the principle of cooperation. We turn next to that principle to reflect on the interface between this theologically substantive vision of Catholic identity and the theological foundations for cooperation.

QUESTIONS FOR REFLECTION AND DISCUSSION

1. In relationship to Catholic health care, the term "charity" can become monetized and refer primarily to charity care or uncompensated care or "caring for the poor." What is the meaning of *caritas* (charity) at the heart of Catholic health care?

2. How does the concrete practice of love in the health care ministry lead to a revelation of God's essence and true nature?

3. How might the different emerging models of health care delivery be able to express *caritas?* Are some models better designed to be in communion with Catholic health care entities?

---

70. See Vatican Council II, *Dei Verbum.*

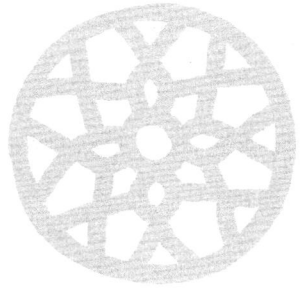

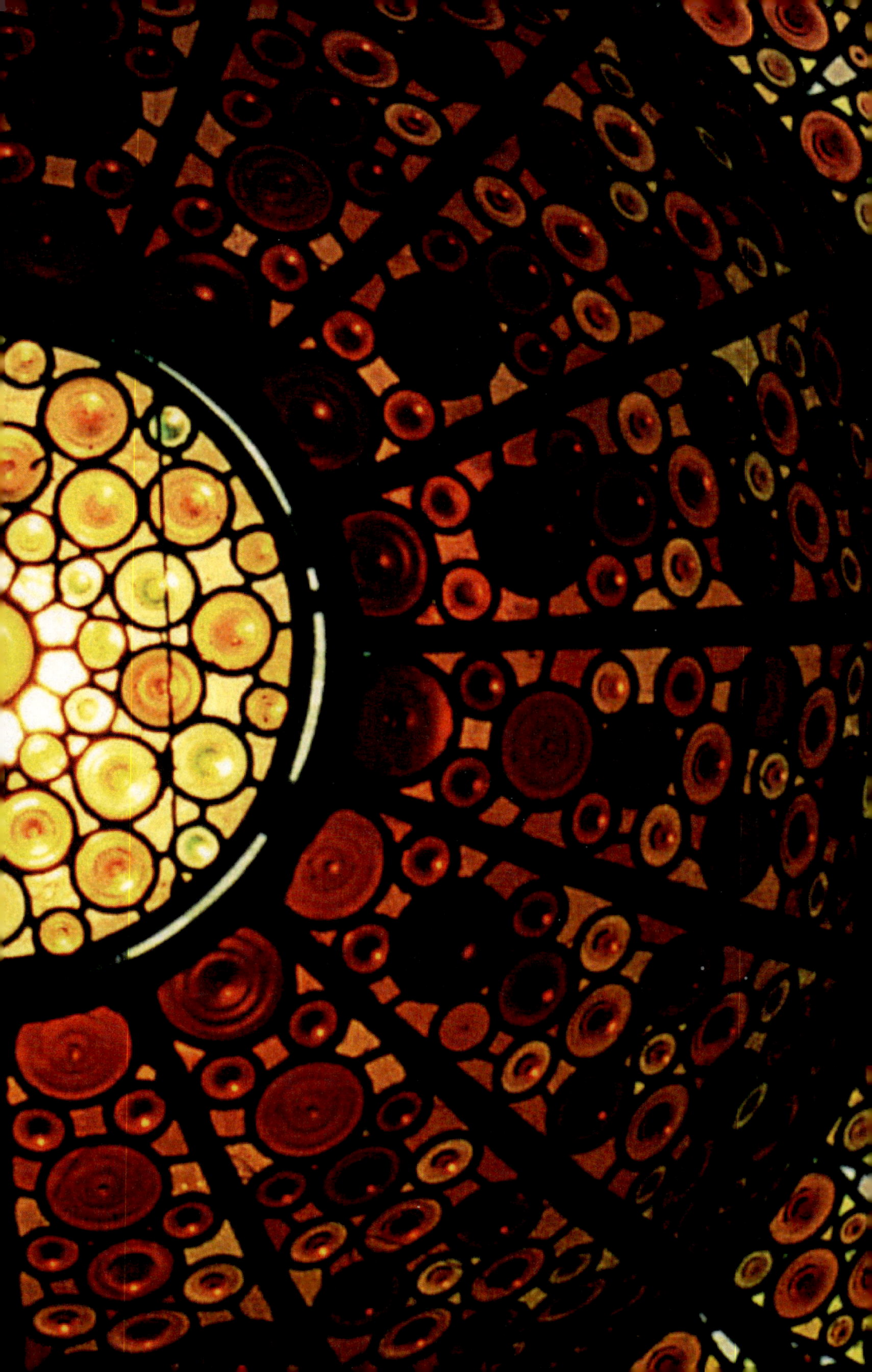

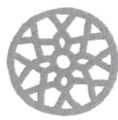

BUILT UPON THESE RICH THEOLOGICAL foundations, Catholic health care is called to be a powerful vehicle of grace in the world. Empowered by the Spirit, Catholic health care has both the privilege and responsibility to live health care in a distinctive way—to demonstrate what health care looks like when shaped on all levels by *caritas* in communion.

This vision, of course, is aspirational. Living *caritas*, whether as individuals or institutions, is a goal we are always moving toward, always seeking to embody in more complete ways. The mundane realities of providing health care in today's market context present significant challenges. As the extensive literature behind the preceding section makes clear, many within Catholic health care have found it challenging to maintain Catholic identity within the traditional Catholic, not-for-profit structures adopted to date. How might the emerging models complicate these challenges? Will it be possible to maintain a richly integrated Catholic identity under secular ownership and management? What new challenges do these arrangements pose?

Consider, for example, the first model outlined in Part II—in which a secular venture capital firm acquires a Catholic hospital. Catholic hospitals purchased by venture funds generally become one investment in a wide-ranging, diversified portfolio. What if other holdings within that portfolio are businesses or industries deeply at odds with Catholic social or moral teaching—arms manufacturers, pharmaceutical companies that manufacture contraceptives, corporations that directly or indirectly sustain sweatshops?[71] What, if any, would be the implications for Catholic identity for the Catholic hospital? Certainly, a venture firm could own socially responsible or socially neutral investments. But portfolios frequently change holdings, and there is no guarantee that a parent company would not acquire companies at odds with Catholic convictions. How ought Catholic hospitals or systems assess these questions as part of the due diligence process? What options do they have if, down the line, the moral complexion of the investment portfolio in which they are included changes?

Alternatively, what might be the implications for a Catholic hospital acquired by a publically traded health care company, especially one with ethically dubious management practices?[72] Will companies that skirt basic ethical and legal regulations permit the Catholic hospitals in their portfolio to shape their internal and external practices according to *caritas*? Or will the practices and commitments of the owner "trickle down" to its managed Catholic hospitals?

71. See, for example, Mark Thompson, "Cerebus To Sell Gun Manufacturer after Massacre," *CNN Money*, December 18, 2012. money.cnn.com/2012/12/18/news/cerberusbushmaster/index.html.

72. Julie Creswell and Reed Abelson, "HCA Discloses U.S. Inquiry into Cardiology Services," *New York Times*, August 6, 2012; Julie Creswell and Reed Abelson, "Giant Hospital Chain Is Blazing a Profit Trail," *New York Times*, August 14, 2012. And the accompanying graphic: http://www.nytimes.com/interactive/2012/08/14/business/HCAs-Growing-Profit.html.

4.1. THE PRINCIPLE OF COOPERATION

For Catholic hospitals, such questions are relatively new. When Catholic hospitals were either stand-alone institutions or parts of systems fully owned and sponsored by religious communities, issues of institutional cooperation were negligible. In recent decades, however, Catholic health care ethicists have found it necessary to analyze the ethical implications of partnerships between Catholic and other-than-Catholic organizations by means of the principle of cooperation, asking whether such ventures may involve formal cooperation or illicit forms of material cooperation on the part of the Catholic partner.[73] In fact, as Catholic health care ethicist John A. Gallagher, Ph.D., notes, since the adoption of the 4TH edition of the *Directives* by the USCCB in 1995, the principle of cooperation has become the primary lens through which potential partnerships are assessed.[74] While this principle has undoubtedly assisted Catholic health institutions and systems in maintaining their identity in a variety of ways, closer reflection upon the principle raises concerns regarding the principle itself and its use in assessing health care partnerships.

In the first place, the principle was originally developed within the context of the practice of confession, as an aid to help individuals determine whether and how they might continue to act morally when they came in contact with or apparently contributed to the actions of others who were involved in wrongdoing.[75] Although the principle was initially applied to the actions of individuals, it has increasingly been used to evaluate the actions of institutions. When applied to institutions, however, the principle is being used analogously.[76]

---

73. See, for example, Ron Hamel, "Cooperation: A Principle that Reflects Reality," *Health Progress* 93, no. 5 (September-October 2012): 80-82.

74. John A. Gallagher, "A Theological Reflection on the Principle of Cooperation and the Catholic Health Ministry," *Health Care Ethics* USA 21, no. 1 (Winter 2013): 2.

75. See Tomas Sanchez, *Opus Morale in Praecepta Decalogi*, Cap. I, Liber 7, 8. See also Alphonsus Liguori, *Theologia Moralis*, Book 2, par 43-80.

76. See, for example, Peter J. Cataldo and John M. Haas, "Institutional Cooperation: The ERDs," *Health Progress* 83, no. 6 (November-December 2002): 83.

Applying the principle in an institutional setting thus becomes more complex and ambiguous than with individuals. Institutional characteristics may affect the outcome of the analysis of cooperation in significant ways.

In addition, some moralists have recently expressed the concern that the principle of cooperation might be used to help health care professionals "avoid being caught engaging in flagrant violations of 'Church law' while sailing as close to the wind as possible." They contrast this with a view of the moral life of institutions that "sees life as the pursuit of perfection…the wholehearted commitment to the holy love of God, neighbor and self," which makes one "much more sensitive to the issues of cooperation in evil."[77] They suggest that Catholic institutions become more circumspect regarding the possibility of interpreting the principle of cooperation too broadly, thereby contradicting the church's prophetic witness.

What has often been missing from these recent discussions of the principle of cooperation has been the richer understanding of cooperation that has been part of the church's social tradition, most recently articulated in the writing of Pope Benedict—especially his encyclicals *Deus Caritas Est* and *Caritas in Veritate*. This section of the paper seeks to move the conversation forward by identifying

---

77. Bishop Anthony Fischer, "Cooperation in Evil: Understanding the Issues" in Helen Watt, ed., *Cooperation, Complicity and Conscience: Problems in Healthcare, Science, Law and Public Policy* (London: The Linacre Centre, 2005), 64.

78. Some Catholic moral theologians wish to emphasize a distinction between the way the term "cooperation" is used in the principle of cooperation and the way the term is used in broader magisterial teaching. This school of thought wishes to reserve the term "cooperation" for analyzing the "cooperation" of Catholics in particular immoral actions of others. They wish to label other modes of Catholic interactions with other-than-Catholics as "collaboration." While they would agree that there is a broad theological mandate for Catholics to *collaborate* with others in the world for the common good, they resist using the term *cooperate* to refer to such interactions.

It is the case, however, that the magisterial tradition privileges the term *cooperation* (at least in English translations). While the magisterial tradition does, on occasion, use the term *collaborate*, it more often uses the term *cooperate*. In addition, while the broader magisterial tradition does not often employ the specific terminology of the principle of cooperation in its broader discussions of Catholic social involvement (e.g., formal, mediate material, and so forth), the shape and logic of the discussions often reflects the conceptual structure of the principle. This study seeks to emphasize the *connections* between the two uses of the term *cooperation* rather than to emphasize their differences. A fuller justification of this approach requires a more academic venue than is available here.

starting points for situating the issue of membership within the broader theological framework of the church's social tradition and its understanding of cooperation.[78] A complete theological foundation for cooperation is beyond the scope of this study and will require further theological development. Here we provide a first step.

4.2. A THEOLOGY OF COOPERATION

One question that arises with regard to the principle of cooperation is whether Christians have a positive obligation to creatively cooperate with others in the world for the common good. Beginning with *Rerum Novarum*, papal commitment to cooperation between Catholics and others for the purpose of advancing the common good grows almost exponentially, reaching its fullest discussion in Pope Benedict's final encyclical, *Caritas in Veritate*. In this section, we trace this tradition and identify the theological grounding of the positive obligation to cooperate.

4.2.1 MAGISTERIAL TRADITION

Papal exhortations toward cooperation emerge as early as *Rerum Novarum* in 1891. Prior to Vatican II, the main issues surrounding cooperation were ecclesiological and ecumenical. May the church cooperate with the state? May Catholics cooperate with other-than-Catholic organizations without "compromising the Catholic unity of the church?"[79] Against opposing voices, the cooperation of Catholics with civic entities and persons of other faith traditions for the common good receives strong papal endorsement. Catholic participation in interfaith activities (such as prayer services) and the ecumenical movement, however, was forbidden as sinful, as it "would imply in the concrete a negation of the Catholic Unity of the Church as a reality already 'given.'"[80]

---

79. John Courtney Murray, "Intercredal Cooperation: Its Theory and Its Organization," *Theological Studies* 4, no. 2 (June 1,1943): 258.

With Vatican II, persons of other faith traditions are no longer described as "wrongdoers."[81] At the same time, Vatican II ratifies the growing commitment of 20TH century papal teaching to the church's vocation to cooperate with the world. As we read in *Gaudium et Spes*:

> Therefore, to encourage and stimulate cooperation among men, the Church must be clearly present in the midst of the community of nations both through her official channels and through the full and sincere collaboration of all Christians— a collaboration motivated solely by the desire to be of service to all (§89).

This commitment to cooperation resounds throughout the writings of Popes Paul, John Paul II, and, most especially, Benedict XVI.[82] We find it frequently in his papal addresses and most notably in *Caritas in Veritate* (2009). Here Pope Benedict continues and develops the longstanding commitment in papal teaching to the cooperation between Catholics and others for the common good, identifying the "urgent need for *new forms* of cooperation at the international, as well as the local level."[83] He names a number of impediments to

---

80. Murray, 257-86. See also Murray, "Cooperation: Some Current Views," *Theological Studies* 4, no. 1 (March 1, 1943): 100-11; and Wilfrid Parsons, "Intercredal Cooperation in the Papal Documents," *Theological Studies* 4, no. 2 (June 1, 1943): 159-82. Secular cultural intellectual Paul Blanshard castigates the Catholic Church for its refusal to permit interfaith cooperation in "The Catholic Price for Cooperation," *Christian Century* 66, no. 18 (May 4, 1949): 557-9. Blanshard's article makes clear that, as late as 1949, many clerics, Catholics, canon law and the moral manuals had not caught up with papal teaching on intercredal cooperation. Notably, the term used almost exclusively in this literature is *cooperation*; the term *collaboration* rarely appears. Moreover, the determination of what is permitted or not, in terms of intercredal cooperation particularly, follows the logic of the terms formal and material as employed by the principle of cooperation. Murray and Parsons would have been familiar with the moral manuals and, therefore, with the principle of cooperation.

81. Second Vatican Council, Decree on Ecumenism (*Unitatis Redintegratio*), and Declaration on the Relation of the Church with Non-Christian Religions (*Nostra Aetate*).

82. For just a few examples, see Pope Benedict XVI, "A New Spirit of Cooperation and Trust," *Osservatore Romano*, 2239: 10/11 (March 28 2012); "Dialogue and Fraternal Cooperation on the Way Toward Unity," *Osservatore Romano* (weekly edition in English), 2148: 6 (June 9 2010); "Religion and Culture for Cooperation between Peoples," *Osservatore Romano* (weekly edition in English), 2145: 6 (May 19 2010); et passim. Again, Pope Benedict heavily favors the term *cooperation*, with *collaboration* coming in a distant second. While this could certainly be an artifact of translation, the ways in which the term is used in these writings provides the stronger argument for connecting the principle of cooperation with this broader context.

83. *Caritas in Veritate*, §25, emphasis added; see also §§61 62, 67, etc.

"the dynamics of cooperation," including technological reductionism (§32) and lack of transparency (§47). Positive cooperation is a form of solidarity and respects subsidiarity (§47).

These explicit references to cooperation as well as the various ways that Pope Benedict articulates this commitment throughout the beginning of the encyclical culminate in the fifth chapter of the encyclical entitled "The Cooperation of the Human Family."[84] His account of cooperation here is deeply theological. At the end of the first paragraph of this chapter he makes clear that Catholics are called beyond a positive obligation to *cooperate* to *communion* with others:

> Today humanity appears much more interactive than in the past: this shared sense of being close to one another must be transformed into true communion. *The development of peoples depends, above all, on a recognition that the human race is a single family* working together in true communion, not simply a group of subjects who happen to live side by side.[85] Pope Paul noted that "the world is in trouble because of the lack of thinking." He was making an observation, but also expressing a wish: a new trajectory of thinking is needed in order to arrive at a better understanding of the implications of our being one family; interaction among the peoples of the world calls us to embark upon this new trajectory, so that integration can signify solidarity rather than marginalization. Thinking of this kind requires *a deeper critical evaluation of the category of relation.*[86]

Cooperative relationships, in Pope Benedict's vision, imply mutuality, a mutuality he sees refused by both secularism and fundamentalism: "Secularism and fundamentalism exclude the possibility of fruitful

---

84. Notably, one sixth of the encyclical focuses on the topic of " cooperation."

85. Here he is citing Pope John Paul, *Evangelium Vitae*, §20: 422-424, emphasis in original.

86. *Caritas in Veritate*, §53, emphasis in original.

dialogue and effective cooperation between reason and religious faith. *Reason always stands in need of being purified by faith:* this also holds true for political reason, which must not consider itself omnipotent. For its part, *religion always needs to be purified by reason* in order to show its authentically human face. Any breach in this dialogue comes only at an enormous price to human development."[87]

Key to his vision is collaboration between believers and non-believers: "Fruitful dialogue between faith and reason cannot but render the work of charity more effective within society, and it constitutes the most appropriate framework for promoting *fraternal collaboration between believers and non-believers* in their shared commitment to working for justice and the peace of the human family."[88]

4.2.2 THEOLOGICAL GROUNDING OF COOPERATION

Pope Benedict's latter comment points to the primary theological grounding for this mandate—again, the theological doctrine of charity. The principle of cooperation is often connected to charity. As Cataldo and Haas note:

> The traditional manuals of Catholic theology have always treated the principle of cooperation in relation to charity. The reasons for this begin with the fact that charity includes acts of "fraternal correction," that is, acts aimed at helping one's neighbor become virtuous. However, insofar as assisting the evil act of a principal agent is contrary to charity (as moral or spiritual correction), it ought to be avoided to the extent possible under the circumstances; this is what the principle of cooperation is designed to do.[89]

---

87. *Caritas in Veritate*, §56, emphasis in original.

88. *Caritas in Veritate*, §57, emphasis in original.

89. Peter J. Cataldo and John M. Haas, "Institutional Cooperation: The ERDs" *Health Progress* 83, no. 6 (November-December 2002): 49-50.

The magisterium also grounds the positive mandate to cooperate in the notion of charity.[90] As a mid-century theologian notes regarding papal writings:

> …several things are immediately manifest. The common effort is in the temporal order—that is its field; the grounds of cooperation are our common membership in the race of men, the one family of the one Father; the cooperation is a duty, and its motive is the law of charity promulgated in the Gospel.[91]

Similarly eminent theologian Fr. John Courtney Murray, SJ, STD, in commenting on a particular papal document, notes:

> It is noteworthy that the Pope recognized the plan as the expression of an impulse of Christian charity, and a desire for a Christian thing—abiding peace in human society, based on the principles of Christian brotherhood. It is still more noteworthy that he viewed the united activity of Christians in the temporal order, animated by a spirit of love, as per se a preparation for the perfect religious unity of the "one flock and one shepherd," which is the will of Christ. We may see two principles here. The first is to take ideas at their best, and give them not only respect but positive welcome, even while we recognize the defect in their inspiration.…The second principle is to acknowledge the genuine unitive value (at least in a preliminary sense) that attaches *per se* to a common exercise of Christian love.[92]

---

90. See, for example, *Rerum Novarum*, §63; *Quadragesimo Anno*, §137, and more.

91. Parsons, 166-7, see also pp. 181-182. He continues: "Less than a year later, Pius XI cleared away any doubt that this passage might have left as to the meaning of 'God's family.' To him it meant the whole human race, not merely the members of the Church; for in his Encyclical *Caritate Christi Impulsi*… broadened the scope of cooperation with men of good will and made it include more constructive aims in the temporal order; he also defined more clearly the reasons that made it necessary [namely, that it was equally a spiritual matter]….His successor, Pius XII, who had been so close to him, lost no time in sounding the same note" (167, 169).

Almost 70 years later, Pope Benedict confirms the connection between cooperation and charity by locating his extensive discussion of cooperation within his encyclical entitled *Caritas in Veritate*. *Caritas in Veritate* also continues the tradition of grounding cooperation in additional theological commitments—theological anthropology, ministry and evangelization, Catholic social teaching, the goodness of God's creation. It is premised on the natural unity of the human family (§55). For Pope Benedict, the *communion* and *relation* between all members of the human family both grounds and is advanced by cooperation. At all points, the purpose of cooperation is to advance the common good—human development, abiding peace in human society, and so forth. Equally, it must be shaped by subsidiarity: "A particular manifestation of charity and a guiding criterion for fraternal cooperation between believers and non-believers is undoubtedly *the principle of subsidiarity*, an expression of inalienable human freedom" (§57). And the common good is advanced in no small part by bringing the love witnessed in the Gospel into the temporal order.

Theological commitments to the goodness of God's creation require a positive understanding of the relationship between the church and the world, and this we find in Pope Benedict's many exhortations toward cooperation. Here he echoes the vision of *Gaudium et Spes*: "[T]he Church seeks but a solitary goal: to carry forward the work of Christ Himself under the lead of the befriending Spirit. And Christ entered this world to give witness to the truth, to rescue and not to sit in judgment, to serve and not to be served" (§3). Cardinal Bernardin,

---

92. Murray, "Cooperation," p. 103. Fr. Murray further notes: "the Catholic concept of cooperation views it indeed as a *co-operatio in caritate* (understanding that duties of the natural order are embraced in the precept of charity), which, however, involves no share in the 'faith' just described for it is of Catholic faith that Christian unity—which is the unity of the world—already exists, a mystical reality embodied in visible form, a Body and a Soul, with all the necessary means for its preservation, its functioning, its growth to all-inclusiveness" (107). The "faith" just described" refers to Murray's interpretation of Protestant positions that cooperation between Catholics and other-than-Catholics implies a unity between denominations, a *co-operatio in fide*. This latter form of cooperation is not permitted, by the magisterium or by Murray, following the logic of formal and material cooperation in wrongdoing (in this case, with wrong belief).

in his 1991 address mentioned earlier, elaborates on this, in a passage that is deeply resonant with *Caritas in Veritate:*

> The church is a community of Jesus' disciples in the midst of the human family. At the same time, the council acknowledged that there is a legitimate secularity in the political, social, and economic orders…[At the Council] a growing awareness developed that the Holy Spirit's influence extends well beyond the confines of the Christian flock to the entire world. This did not take away from the truth which the church teaches, but it opened the church to the possibility of discovering elements of the truth which others possess, even as it brings the message of the Gospel to the world, even as it provides a moral and ethical framework in which societal issues can be evaluated and challenged. The *Pastoral Constitution on the Church in the Modern World* states that the church has much to learn from the world. The world is a possible partner for dialogue, a mutual exchange. While we may take this for granted at least on a theological level, it was not always the thinking of the church or its members; nor do we yet have sufficient experience or expertise to carry on such a dialogue in a way that will realize its full potential….[93]

Neither Pope Benedict nor Cardinal Bernardin are naïve or uncritical about the world, but as the latter notes "neither should we be too quick to reject or distrust the world. If our participation in the dialogue is not an accommodation to the world but rather that truth, spoken in love, we need not fear that dialogue will jeopardize or dilute the prophetic, countercultural message of the Gospel."[94]

---

93. Bernardin, 1991. See also Skylstad, 92.

94. Bernardin, 1991.

4.2.3 A THEOLOGY OF COOPERATION AND CATHOLIC HEALTH CARE

Thus, Catholic health care finds itself not only *permitted* to enter into partnerships with other faith based and secular organizations; it finds a positive obligation to engage in *"fraternal collaboration between believers and non-believers."*[95] Especially within the U.S., health care remains "an issue of justice and peace" for so many members of the human family. Fraternal collaboration "renders the work of charity more effective."

Pope Benedict's vision of this cooperation is shaped by key terms: dialogue, mutuality, true communion, recognition of each other's personhood, one family, solidarity rather than marginalization, category of relation. It is important that he identifies fundamentalism as a stumbling block to cooperative relationships and recognizes that as much as faith brings to our secular partners, *religion always needs to be purified by reason.*

The primary agents of this cooperation of the human family will be lay persons. As noted earlier, prior to Vatican II, the church lacked a theological account of the laity. Here, as in many cases, however, practice preceded theory. For the 20TH century popes, the agents of cooperation in the world were lay persons, particularly those involved with Catholic Action and other lay Catholic groups (such as Catholic trade unions). Vatican II drew on these decades of lay engagement and initiated what remains an ongoing process of developing a theologically sound understanding of who lay persons are, the sacramental origin of their various ministries, and the relationship between their leadership and authority and that of ecclesial leadership and authority.

Cardinal Bernardin, continuing his reflection on the often-conflicted social location of those in Catholic higher education, social services

---

95. *Caritas in Veritate*, §57, emphasis in original.

and health care, who "work along the fault line of the church's dialogue with the world," recognizes "they are in a privileged position to learn from the world and to share that knowledge and insight with the rest of the community of faith." Equally, they have the responsibility to bring the Gospel to those they encounter in this dialogue. Cardinal Bernardin envisages lay persons as leaders in ministering to the world and advancing the church.

Cardinal Bernardin's insights are echoed 20 years later in an important reflection by Pope Benedict entitled "The Co-Responsibility of the Laity." In a short address to an August 22-26, 2012 gathering of the International Forum of Catholic Action, Pope Benedict clearly endorses a strong vision of lay identity: "All church members need to make a renewed effort to ensure laypeople are aware of their responsibility for the church and are allowed to exercise it....Co-responsibility demands a change in mind-set, especially concerning the role of lay people in the church. They should not be regarded as 'collaborators' of the clergy but rather as people who are really 'co-responsible' for the church's being and acting." Drawing on *Lumen Gentium*, he notes that "Viewing the church as a family emphasizes shared responsibility, mutual support, and joint action while, at the same time, recognizing the special role of guidance belonging to the church's pastors" (254). Further, such joint action must respect the legitimate autonomy and respective competences of those with whom we cooperate.[96]

4.4 CONCLUSION

This, then, is a first component of the broader theological context within which Catholic partnerships should be interpreted and applied. Rooted in the unity of the human family; a positive vision of church/world state; an increasing appreciation of the co-responsibility of the laity for the church; and charity, we find the beginnings of a richly grounded theology of cooperation. Again, we can identify

---

96. *Deus Caritas Est*, §29.

this theological foundation as *caritas* in communion. This theology suggests not, primarily, that fraternal cooperation with other-than-Catholics complicates efforts to maintain Catholic identity; it suggests that it is, in fact, an important manifestation of the theological foundations of Catholic identity. It is, moreover, one component of the legitimate moral and theological authority that accompanies lay persons' sacramental vocation, the practical experience and real knowledge and insight that comes from their constant negotiation of the "fault line," and their lived practice of discipleship.

Moreover, cooperation between Catholics and other-than-Catholics can bear rich fruit for the Gospel and human development in society. In addition to the critical work of delivering health care across populations, especially to the poor and marginalized, in most of their partnerships, Catholic systems have been remarkably successful in influencing other institutions to adopt many Catholic values. The success of Catholic systems in achieving this level of *practical* moral consensus appears to be without parallel in the U.S. context. It is also largely unrecognized and unlauded.

These positive effects of Catholic partnerships with other-than-Catholics reinforce Fr. Morrisey's call for a new dialogue around the principle of cooperation mentioned earlier—to orient our discussions away from a narrow focus on direct sterilization toward the overall mission of Catholic health care which is the mission of Christ. Echoing the foregoing analysis, Fr. Morrisey cites the conceptual shift surrounding ecumenism that came with Vatican II, noting that while there are certainly "'messy'" areas that have to be addressed — inter-communion and ordination being two of them…these obstacles did not prevent the church from moving forward with dialogue and many concrete acts of ecumenism,"[97] that have greatly advanced the work of the Kingdom of God in the world.

---

97. Morrisey, 2013, p. 66.

This analysis, therefore, articulates a broader context for considering new forms of partnerships. This approach seeks to align conversations around cooperation with developments in papal social theory and ecumenism—seeing the cooperative, collaborative work of Catholics with others toward the goods we hold in common as more determinative than ongoing areas of disagreement. It challenges those who interpret the principle of cooperation to more adequately conceptualize the collaboration of institutional agents in the social sphere rather than employing a method designed for individual agents in the personal sphere. It seeks to expand the context of considerations around cooperation beyond simply material cooperation in reproductive acts to broader issues such as the ways potential partnerships may draw Catholic organizations into structures of sin.[98] It seeks to integrate the principle of cooperation with the principles of Catholic social thought, particularly in relationship to the promotion of the common good and the proper subsidiarity of other-than-Catholic partners.

For it may well be that some of the emerging models of partnership might, via the principle of subsidiarity, provide a more appropriate space for fraternal cooperation. If other-than-Catholic (secular) not-for-profit parent organizations are structured so as to allow all participants their proper subsidiarity, they may well prove amenable to the maintenance of Catholic identity within hospitals and subsystems. They may allow for a greater range of Catholic partnerships with other faith-based or secular providers of health care, increasing the scope of the work of charity in the world.

Partnership is one form of dialogue. The main question is: does the structure of a proposed organization—especially where one

---

98. This broader theology of cooperation does not suggest that questions of cooperating in "evil acts" is no longer relevant. It does suggest that analyses of such acts must include more considerations than simply the distinctions embedded in the principle (formal, material, etc.). It also suggests that of equal concern for Catholic health care institutions are not occasional immoral acts of individuals but rather the "structures of sin" first identified by Pope John Paul II, which are more pressing realities for a ministry like Catholic health care. The principle of cooperation provides few resources for thinking about the participation of Catholics or Catholic institutions in structures of sin.

party is managed by the other—diminish the mutuality necessary for dialogue and true collaboration? In the next section, we turn to Catholic social teaching to address this question. As we will see, the answers to the questions raised in this study are less a matter of "yes" or "no" than they are questions of *how*. Structures do matter. How these relationships are structured will go a long way toward ensuring that Catholic participants have the necessary freedom and material support to continue to integrate Catholic identity into their hospitals and systems. They may also provide Catholic hospitals and systems with an impetus to more intentionally and concretely integrate Catholic commitments into their internal structures.

QUESTIONS FOR REFLECTION AND DISCUSSION

1. This study distinguishes the principle of cooperation used in Catholic moral theology from a larger theology of cooperation or collaboration. Is this distinction helpful in addressing the challenges that arise from the current organization of Catholic health care?

2. Since fraternal collaboration (with other faith based and secular organizations) can render the work of charity more effective, how might Catholic health care organizations ethically pursue such work in order to serve the common good?

3. How might collaborative structures be built so that Catholic participants have the necessary freedom and material support to continue to integrate Catholic identity into their hospitals and systems?

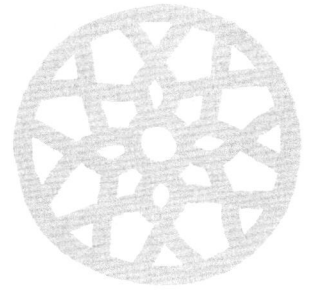

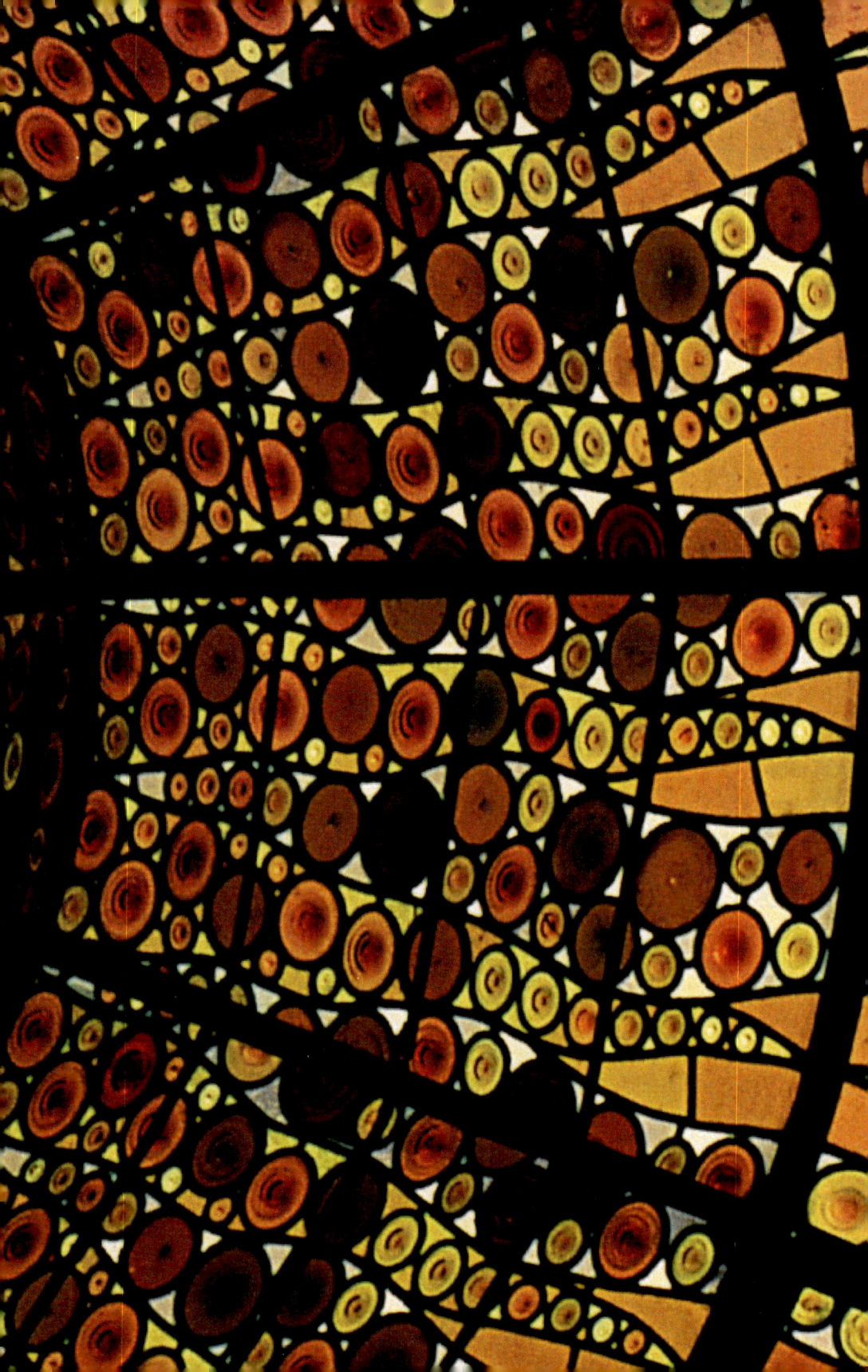

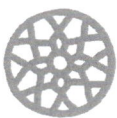

V. THEOLOGICAL FOUNDATIONS OF CATHOLIC ECONOMIC THOUGHT: THE FOR-PROFIT QUESTION

S R. DORIS GOTTEMOELLER, RSM, PH.D., NOTES "there is no authoritative doctrinal teaching" on the question of whether Catholic ministries, particularly health care organizations, ought to adopt for-profit or not-for-profit corporate status, as these terms are defined in the U.S. context.[99] Nor has the question received attention from the theological disciplines.

Therefore, this study provides an outline of the theological parameters for discernment around the question of for-profit corporate status for Catholic health care organizations. From a practical perspective, this is an extraordinarily complex question. For the purposes of the CHA membership study, the question under consideration is whether the shift from not-for-profit corporate status to for-profit status by systems or hospitals is consistent with Catholic identity. However, over the past two decades, most Catholic systems have adopted or created one or more for-profit subsidiaries within their overall organization. The reasons for this are usually driven by state law, such

---

99. Gottemoeller, "For Profit and Catholic? How Would the Ministry Fare?" *Health Progress* 93, no.4 (July-August 2012): 31.

as the corporate practice of medicine or the need to enter into joint venture arrangements with for-profit partners. In some cases, the for-profit subsidiary is wholly owned by a not-for-profit Catholic entity; in other cases, the Catholic not-for-profit entity is a majority owner in a for-profit joint venture with a for-profit partner; in yet other cases, the Catholic not-for-profit entity is a minority owner in a for-profit joint venture with a for-profit partner. In addition, Catholic systems may own portfolios of investments, thereby participating in the for-profit world in a variety of ways. An increasing percentage of the bottom line for Catholic health systems now derives from such subsidiary for-profit components.

These new developments within Catholic health care have arisen only recently. They have not raised questions for CHA membership, and the ministry as a whole appears to be comfortable with having these sorts of for-profit structures in its midst as long as the ultimate parent company is not-for-profit and can "control" the values of the subsidiaries. Yet these developments have not received careful theological assessment.

Such an assessment is beyond the scope of this white paper, which will focus primarily on the question of the for-profit/not-for-profit status of a "parent" organization in a Catholic health care system or a Catholic hospital. This paper will attempt to keep focused on the question driving the discernment around the question of membership: whether, in a publicly traded structure or a privately held structure with a venture capital firm, values central to Catholic identity are more likely to be compromised or more difficult to uphold than they would be under a not-for-profit parent structure.

A thorough theological analysis of the foregoing questions would include careful attention to: the history of economics, especially over the past 300 years; the emerging discipline of theological economics; scriptural insights regarding the relationship between economics and Judeo-Christian discipleship; as well as magisterial teaching on economic and social questions. Unfortunately, such a careful study is beyond the scope of this paper. Therefore, the following section will focus primarily on the parameters given within magisterial teaching on economics and social questions, as found in the corpus of Catholic social thought.

Behind these principles lie fundamental theological commitments. By now, it should come as no surprise that a central theological foundation for Catholic economic thought is *caritas*—here articulated by Pope Benedict as the *principle of gratuitousness*. Equally critical are doctrines of the human person (specifically, the dignity of workers and integral human development) and creation (a vision of property) integrated through the lens of communion (solidarity). These theological commitments shape a distinctive Catholic vision of the business enterprise that provides a helpful framework for evaluating the question of the fit between for-profit corporate structures and Catholic identity, a framework that can again be summed up in the phrase *caritas* in communion.

5.1 WHAT DO WE MEAN BY "FOR-PROFIT"?

Before analyzing the question of "for-profit" corporate status, it is necessary to clarify the term "for-profit." "For-profit" in this analysis does *not* refer to the following. It does not refer to the simple process of "revenue over expenses." All business, service or ministerial enterprises must find themselves (at least more often than not) "in the black." Through a variety of income sources (revenues, donations, grants, etc.) combined with prudential expenditure, all incorporated enterprises should realize a net of revenue over expenses or else they will cease to exist. Catholic health care institutions—even those that have not-for-profit corporate status—clearly must "make a profit" in this sense. Similarly, the term "for-profit" does *not* refer to the fact that individuals—such as individual physicians—earn an income or "profit" from delivering health care services in their physician practices. Although some do question the amount of income some physicians make, such income should be understood as remuneration for work provided rather than "profit" in the technical sense discussed below.

At issue is the precise nature of "for-profit" corporate structures as they function in the United States, both legally and culturally. A for-profit corporation is a corporation that is, by definition, intended to return a portion of surplus revenues to owners or investors. It may be operated either as a stock corporation or as a non-stock corporation. It may be publicly traded or privately held. A not-for-profit corporation is a corporation that, by definition, cannot distribute surplus revenues as profits or dividends to owners or investors, but rather must use surplus revenues to achieve other specified goals. These goals include preserving or expanding the corporation itself or funding community goods.[100]

Thus, a first question is: where do profits go? Do they go to the community, to the corporation itself, or to individuals? What ends do they serve? Do they serve community goods? Do they serve to build up the company itself? Or do they serve the private ends of individuals? These are important questions for Catholic health care because within the Catholic tradition, the morality of actions and institutions is determined in part by their "ends," by the goods or goals they seek and realize.

A second question is also "end" oriented. It is the question: in a for-profit corporate structure will "profit" become the main end or goal of the organization, to the detriment of other important ends, goods or goals? This appears to be one of the main concerns voiced by many who work in Catholic health care with regard to the shift from not-for-profit to for-profit corporate status. These concerns center on what is known as the principle of "shareholder primacy." The

---

100. The terms "for-profit" and "not-for-profit"/"non-profit" are state law concepts and do not in and of themselves connote tax status. Under federal tax law, all corporations, whether organized as for-profit or not-for-profit under state law, are considered taxable entities, unless granted tax-exempt status under federal law. An entity must be not-for-profit to qualify for federal tax-exempt status, but not all not-for-profits are necessarily tax exempt.

principle of shareholder primacy holds that for-profit companies are obligated to make profit-for-owners/investors a primary end to which all other ends are secondary.[101] In other words, there is a cultural assumption that for-profit companies are obliged to maximize profits for the sake of shareholders.

This assumption is widely held culturally[102] and is taught almost universally in business schools.[103] It derives from a precedent-setting case, Dodge v. Ford (1919), that stated:

> There should be no confusion . . . . A business corporation is organized and carried on primarily for the profit of the stockholders. The powers of the directors are to be employed for that end. The discretion of the directors is to be exercised in the choice of means to attain that end, and does not extend to . . . other purposes.[104]

Subsequent case law regarding corporate profits has followed this line of reasoning.[105] It is also presumed in the American Law Institute's

---

101. Judd F. Sneirson, "The Sustainable Corporation and Shareholder Profits," *Wake Forest Law Review* 46 (2011): 541-559 at 548.

102. Certain economists have been very effective in communicating these assumptions within public media and thereby shaping cultural consciousness. See, as a classic example, Milton Friedman's, "The Social Responsibility of Business Is To Increase Its Profits," *New York Times Magazine*, September 13, 1970. For a critical examination of the cultural power of this assumption, see Joel Bakan's, *The Corporation: The Pathological Pursuit of Profit and Power* (New York: Free Press, 2005); as well as the documentary by the same title. Michael Troilo notes that Helen Alford and Michael Naughton "maintain that the discipline of finance has moved beyond a technique for profit maximization into a social philosophy that establishes profits as the chief end in and of itself," (Michael Louis Troilo, "*Caritas in Veritate*, Hybrid Firms, and Institutional Arrangements," *Journal of Markets & Morality* 14, no. 1 (March 1, 2011): 26).

103. See Lynn Stout, "Why We Should Stop Teaching Dodge v. Ford," *Virginia Law and Business Review* 3.1 (2008): 164-176; and Jonathan R. Macey, "A Close Read of an Excellent Commentary on Dodge v Ford," *Virginia Law and Business Review*, 3, no. 1 (Spring 2008): 177-190. For example, the online *Business Dictionary* defines a for-profit organization as: "A business or other organization whose primary goal is making money (a profit), as opposed to a non-profit organization which focuses a goal such as helping the community and is concerned with money only as much as necessary to keep the organization operating." See: http://www.businessdictionary.com/definition/for-profit-organization. html#ixzz2ONW0SUyz.

104. Cited in Stout, 165.

105. Stout, 169; Sneirson, 550-1; Macey, 178. Einer Elhuge refers to this as "the canonical account" ("Sacrificing Corporate Profits in the Public Interest," presentation at Harvard University, 2003, p. 1).

(ALI) *Principles of Corporate Governance*, which is considered "a significant, if not controlling, source of doctrinal authority."[106] As Jonathan Macey, JD, notes: "specifically, section 2.01 of the *Principles* makes clear that 'a corporation should have as its objective the conduct of business activities with a view to enhancing corporate profit and shareholder gain'...[and they] specify that the goal of the corporation is shareholder wealth maximization."[107]

At the same time, scholars of law and economics currently debate whether there is in fact an actual "legal proposition that a corporation must maximize shareholder profits."[108] Recent opinion suggests that pursuit of humanitarian, charitable, social or other-stakeholder objectives is within the discretion of corporate leadership.[109] The ALI *Principles* cited above contain "three rather minor exceptions to the shareholder wealth maximization norm. Corporations can ignore shareholder wealth maximization in order to: (1) comply with the law; (2) make charitable contributions; and (3) devote a 'reasonable amount of resources to public welfare, humanitarian, educational, and philanthropic purposes.'"[110]

Nonetheless, scholarly consensus holds that even if the obligation to *maximize* profit for shareholders/owners is not legally binding, and if other ends can be legitimately pursued within a for-profit structure, they can be pursued only as long as owner/shareholder profits are to some degree *enhanced*.[111] In other words, corporate law remains "shareholder-centric" and the principle of shareholder primacy is subtly operative.[112] Moreover, as Judd Sneirson, JD, notes: "Even

---

106. Macey, 178. See also Sneirson, 552.

107. Macey, 178.

108. Stout, 168; Sneirson, 550.

109. Stout, 168; Elhuge.

110. Macey, 178-9; Elhuge, 7. Elhuge notes that corporate law appears to limit such pursuits to no more than 10 per cent of corporate tax income (7).

111. Sneierson, 552.

112. Sneirson, 550 or 551.

if no law requires shareholder primacy, a prevalent social norm can have much the same effect."[113] Therefore, the concern voiced by many within Catholic health care—that a shift to a for-profit corporate structure may render the end of health care delivery secondary to the end of profits-for-investors—is a valid concern.

5.2　KEY COMMITMENTS OF CATHOLIC SOCIAL DOCTRINE

A first step in analyzing the fit between for-profit corporate structures as described above and Catholic identity is to locate the question within the context of Catholic social doctrine. A review of this literature provides five principles or commitments that are relevant to the question of for-profit status. These are: the notion of integral human development, the dignity and priority of labor, structures of sin and solidarity, private property and the universal destination of goods, and the principle of gratuitousness.

5.2.1　INTEGRAL HUMAN DEVELOPMENT

From *Rerum Novarum* forward, papal teaching on economic questions has emphasized that just economic systems must attend to more than simply wages. Pope Paul, concerned that international organizations were attending solely to questions of economic development, coins a new phrase in *Populorum Progressio*—integral human development. For Pope Paul and his successors, integral human development captures the tradition's attention to the dignity of the whole human person and emphasizes that economic progress must be sought in conjunction with and subordinated to other goods critical for the full flourishing of human persons in community— physical, spiritual, emotional, psychological, social and familial goods. Only integral human development helps persons move toward fulfillment of their individual gifts and capacities, and, in so doing, promotes the flourishing of the common good. Rather than being a

---

113. Sneirson, 554.

burden on businesses, Pope John Paul specifically maintains that "the integral development of the human person through work does not impede but rather promotes the greater productivity and efficiency of work itself."[114] In many ways, the notion of integral human development also becomes a concept that integrates the multiple principles of Catholic social thought.

5.2.2 THE DIGNITY AND PRIORITY OF LABOR

Pope John Paul's 1981 encyclical *Laborem Exercens*, "On Human Work," commemorates the 90TH anniversary of *Rerum Novarum*.[115] He opens by stating that the question of human work has been at the heart of the church's attention to "the social question" from the very beginning of the tradition (§§2-3). Work is not simply a process by which one earns wages to pay for material goods. It is a central and primary activity by which persons move toward their fulfillment as human persons, by which they advance toward full human flourishing. It engages the essence of the human person and promotes her or his integral development. Thus, Pope John Paul reaffirms the church's position from *Rerum Novarum* forward of "the priority of labor over capital": "In view of this situation we must first of all recall a principle that has always been taught by the Church: the principle of the priority of labour over capital" (§12). Or, as he will say elsewhere repeatedly: "the priority of persons over profit."

This emphasis on the centrality of work continues in *Centesimus Annus*. While *Centesimus Annus* is often read as a celebration of capitalism and wealth creation, even a cursory reading of the document makes clear that Pope John Paul's main focus is the "worker," continuing the focus of *Rerum Novarum* and his own commitment to the dignity of persons as workers articulated in

---

114. Diarmud Martin, "Catholic Social Teaching and Human Work: The 25th Anniversary of *Laborem Exercens*," *Journal of Catholic Social Thought* 6, no. 1 (2009): 11.

115. Pope John Paul II, *Laborem Exercens*, 1981.

Laborem Exercens.[116] For example, he notes in *Centesimus Annus* that "in our time, the role of human work is becoming increasingly important as the productive factor both of non-material and of material wealth. Moreover, it is becoming clearer how a person's work is naturally interrelated with the work of others. More than ever, work is work with others and work for others: it is a matter of doing something for someone else."[117] In other words, Pope John Paul ties work, not capital, to wealth creation.[118]

5.2.3 THE STRUCTURES OF SIN AND SOLIDARITY

In Pope John Paul's encyclical *Sollicitudo Rei Socialis* (1987), he speaks of a "duty of solidarity," for "political leaders and citizens of rich countries" to examine the relationship between their own lives and the world's poverty (§9). At the root of the grave poverty he describes lies what he identifies, for the first time in a papal encyclical, as the "structures of sin": "The sum total of the negative factors working against a true awareness of the universal common good, and the need to further it" (§36). Such structures "are rooted in personal sin, and thus always linked to the concrete acts of individuals who introduce these structures, consolidate them and make them difficult to remove. And thus they grow stronger, spread, and become the source of other sins, and so influence people's behavior" (§36; cf §37).

Pope John Paul very specifically identifies two main, intertwined structures of sin: "*the all-consuming desire for profit*, and … the thirst for power, with the intention of imposing one's will upon others. In order to characterize better each of these attitudes, one can add the expression: 'at any price'.… behind certain decisions, apparently

---

116. See *Centesimus Annus*, §3-6, etc. Moreover, *Centesimus Annus* carries through all the main themes of Catholic social doctrine, including its simultaneous appreciation and critique of capitalist economic structures.

117. *Centesimus Annus*, §31.

118. *Centesimus Annus*, §32, which could be read to refer to capital rather than labor, celebrates the initiative, vision and work of entrepreneurial persons.

inspired only by economics or politics, are real forms of *idolatry: of money*, ideology, class, technology."[119]

The solution to such structures of sin is solidarity. Solidarity, which Pope John Paul names as a "virtue" is:

> a firm and persevering determination to commit oneself to the common good; that is to say to the good of all and of each individual, because we are all really responsible for all. This determination is based on the solid conviction that *what is hindering full development is that desire for profit* and that thirst for power already mentioned. These attitudes and "structures of sin" are only conquered—presupposing the help of divine grace—by a diametrically opposed attitude: a commitment to the good of one's neighbor with the readiness, in the Gospel sense, to "lose oneself" for the sake of the other instead of exploiting him, and to "serve him" instead of oppressing him for one's own advantage (cf. Mt 10:40-42; 20: 25; Mk 10: 42-45; Lk 22: 25-27).[120]

Solidarity—a call to communion—is rooted in the recognition that those oppressed by the structures of sin are human persons whose dignity and integral human development have been ignored and undermined. As will be discussed further below, it is also rooted in charity, not simply almsgiving, but *caritas*.

5.2.4   PRIVATE PROPERTY AND THE UNIVERSAL DESTINATION OF GOODS

The right to private property was established as a key component of the Catholic social tradition with *Rerum Novarum*. Yet, as Pope John Paul notes, Pope Leo "is well aware that private property is

---

119. *Sollicitudo*, §37 (emphasis added).

120. *Sollicitudo*, §38 (emphasis added).

not an absolute value, nor does he fail to proclaim the necessary complementary principles, such as the universal destination of the earth's goods."[121] Similarly, when Pope John Paul discusses private property, he always links it to the universal destination of goods. In fact he notes that "the Successors of Leo XIII have repeated this twofold affirmation: the necessity and therefore the legitimacy of private ownership, as well as the limits which are imposed on it."[122]

The universal destination of goods is an important notion in Catholic economic thought. Articulated by Augustine, Thomas Aquinas, and traced to Genesis, the principle, referenced repeatedly in the Catholic social encyclicals, maintains that, the principle of private property notwithstanding, the goods of creation, gifted to humanity by God, are meant for all, for sustaining human life and well-being. As Pope John Paul states in *Sollicitudo*:

> It is necessary to state once more the characteristic principle of Christian social doctrine: the goods of this world are originally meant for all. The right to private property is valid and necessary, but it does not nullify the value of this principle. Private property, in fact, is under a "social mortgage," which means that it has an intrinsically social function, based upon and justified precisely by the principle of the universal destination of goods (§42).[123]

> Interdependence must be transformed into solidarity, based upon the principle that the goods of creation are meant for all. That which human industry produces through the processing of raw materials, with the contribution of work, must serve equally for the good of all (§39).

---

121. *Centesimus Annus*, §12 and §30.

122. *Centesimus Annus*, §30.

123. See also *Laborem Exercens*, §12; Pope John Paul devotes an entire chapter of *Centesimus Annus* to the relationship between private property and the universal destination of goods (Ch. IV, §30ff).

In other words, the right to private property is always qualified by the basic needs of others—those material goods necessary to maintain human life.[124]

In addition to affirming the universal destination of goods, Pope John Paul also distinguishes between types of goods—those that can be commodified and social goods. Too often the first sentence of the following section is detached from the rest of its paragraph and is taken out of context:

> It would appear that, on the level of individual nations and
> of international relations, the free market is the most efficient
> instrument for utilizing resources and effectively responding
> to needs. But this is true only for those needs which are
> "solvent," insofar as they are endowed with purchasing power,
> and for those resources which are "marketable," insofar as
> they are capable of obtaining a satisfactory price. But there
> are many human needs which find no place on the market. It
> is a strict duty of justice and truth not to allow fundamental
> human needs to remain unsatisfied, and not to allow those
> burdened by such needs to perish....Even prior to the logic of
> a fair exchange of goods and the forms of justice appropriate
> to it, there exists something which is due to man because he
> is man, by reason of his lofty dignity. Inseparable from that
> required "something" is the possibility to survive and, at the
> same time, to make an active contribution to the common
> good of humanity.[125]

Later in *Centesimus Annus* he reaffirms this position:

> Here we find a new limit on the market: there are collective
> and qualitative needs which cannot be satisfied by market

124. See also *Centesimus Annus*, §30.

125. *Centesimus Annus*, §34.

mechanisms. There are important human needs which escape its logic. There are goods which by their very nature cannot and must not be bought or sold. Certainly the mechanisms of the market offer secure advantages: they help to utilize resources better; they promote the exchange of products; above all they give central place to the person's desires and preferences, which, in a contract, meet the desires and preferences of another person. Nevertheless, these mechanisms carry the risk of an "idolatry" of the market, an idolatry which ignores the existence of goods which by their nature are not and cannot be mere commodities.[126]

Although Pope John Paul does not name any particular needs "which find no place in the market," his description of such needs would certainly include health care, insofar as without it, people perish, is required for persons to actively contribute to the common good, and is due to persons simply because of their human dignity.

QUESTIONS FOR REFLECTION AND DISCUSSION

1. Within the Catholic tradition, the morality of actions and institutions is determined in part by their "ends," by the good or goals they seek and realize. With that in mind, what questions should be raised when a Catholic health care entity embarks on the consideration of a collaborative business enterprise with a for-profit organization?

2. How would solidarity be realized in a collaborative relationship between a for-profit business enterprise and a Catholic health care ministry?

---

126. *Centesimus Annus*, §40.

3. The principles of Catholic social thought challenge conventional ways of understanding the business enterprise. How can the principle of gratuitousness exist in the context of conventional economic, social and political practices?

5.2.5 THE PRINCIPLE OF GRATUITOUSNESS

Caritas in Veritate, Pope Benedict's third and most recent encyclical (2009), continues the tradition of *Populorum Progressio*, commenting on international economics from a theological perspective. While sounding many of the same themes as *Populorum Progressio, Sollicitudo Rei Socialis*, and the Catholic social tradition in general, Pope Benedict adds a new principle to the network: what he calls "the principle of gratuitousness." Since it is newly articulated, it merits closer attention.

While charity is central in the Catholic social tradition from *Rerum Novarum* forward, this principle of gratuitousness begins to emerge in the writings of Pope John Paul, as noted above.[127] Pope Benedict develops these earlier hints into a principle in its own right. From the title forward, his encyclical on global economic realities is centered on charity as a theological concept. *Caritas*, as discussed earlier, is at the heart of the church's social doctrine and is the principal driving force behind integral human development. It is necessarily so, he notes, because charity is, in reality, grace, the inner dynamic of love among Persons of the Trinity.

Pope Benedict outlines a series of ways in which God's presence—as absolutely gratuitous gift—"bursts into our lives as something not due to us, something that transcends every law of justice" (§34). Hope, God's very presence to us, the goods of creation, truth, the truth of ourselves, our personal consciences—all these things and more we encounter as *gift*. At the center of all reality—at the reality

---

127. See also *Sollicitudo*, §40.

experienced by each and every person—is the reality of *gift*. From this he concludes that "economic, social, and political development, if it is to be authentically human, needs to make room for the principle of gratuitousness as an expression of fraternity" (emphasis in original, §34). This is no mere individual, tax-benefit earning almsgiving. For Pope Benedict, the principle of gratuitousness ought to shape economic, social and political practices:

> …in *commercial relationships* the *principle of gratuitousness* and the logic of gift as an expression of fraternity can and must *find their place within normal economic activity*. This is a human demand at the present time, but it is also demanded by economic logic. It is a demand of both charity and of truth (emphasis in original, §36).

This principle of gratuitousness does not simply reject contemporary economic practices, but it calls for freedom and creativity within them. As he notes:

> Space also needs to be created within the market for economic activity to be carried out by subjects who freely choose to act according to principles other than those of pure profit, without sacrificing the production of economic value in the process. The many economic entities that draw their origin from religious and lay initiatives demonstrate that this is concretely possible (§37).

Economic life, he acknowledges, requires contracts, just laws and forms of redistribution via politics, but "what is more, it needs works redolent of the *spirit of gift*. The economy in the global era seems to privilege the former logic, that of contractual exchange, but directly or indirectly it also demonstrates its need for the other two: political logic, and the logic of the unconditional gift" (emphasis in original, §37).

For Pope Benedict then, particularly in light of the economic crisis that began in 2007, the principle of gratuitousness must become an intrinsic part of contemporary economic practices. Catholic institutions have a particular obligation to attempt to embody this principle as a way of demonstrating to the wider culture what the logic of gift might look like within contemporary market practices. Catholic health systems, in particular, are called to such a challenge. For the massive reality that is Catholic health care was built on the logic of gift—not only the gift of health care to the poor and the donation of funds from so many faithful Catholics but also the charity/gift of the religious who worked for Catholic hospitals for little or no compensation. The powerful economic reality of Catholic health care today was made by possible by the practice of *caritas*.

5.3 THE BUSINESS ENTERPRISE IN THE CATHOLIC TRADITION

Pope Benedict—and these principles of Catholic social thought generally—challenge conventional ways of understanding the business enterprise. As he notes: "Today's international economic scene, marked by grave deviations and failures, requires a *profoundly new way of understanding business enterprise*" (*Caritas in Veritate*, §40, emphasis in original).

Economist Charles M.A. Clark, Ph.D., makes clear that a fundamental difference between Catholic approaches to economics and secular approaches to economics lies in their understanding of the human person. Inherent in the logic and the philosophy of capitalism, in its unbridled form, is a momentum to reduce persons to "a mere instrument of production."[128] While the Catholic tradition is strongly supportive of business, trade and even capitalist forms of economics, it always sees them as "bridled"—as secondary

128. Charles M.A. Clark, "Economic Life in Catholic Social Thought and Economic Theory" in *Catholic Social Thought: American Reflections on the Compendium*, edited by D. Paul Sullins and Anthony J. Blasi (Lanham, Md.: Lexington Books, 2009) 77-99. And Clark, "Catholic Social Thought and the Economic Problem" *OIKONOMIA*, no. 1, February 2001, pp. 6-18. See also *Centesimus Annus*, §4.

to the dignity of the human person and the promotion of the community/common good, as tools or means for promoting the flourishing of persons and communities.[129]

This leads to a markedly different way of understanding the business enterprise. For Pope John Paul, a business is certainly not the "nexus of contracts" that dominates U.S. corporate theory.[130] Even further, it "cannot be considered only as a 'society of capital goods'; it is, rather, a 'society of persons.'"[131] It is also a "community of work."[132] As such, a corporation is a society of moral agents who work together for the common good, "a community of solidarity that is not closed within its own company interests."[133] As he says elsewhere, "…Christians charged with responsibility in the business world are challenged to combine the legitimate pursuit of profit with a deeper concern for the spread of solidarity and the elimination of the scourge of poverty."[134]

For a Catholic institution, "profit" can never be an end in itself; it is always a secondary good, an instrument for achieving other outcomes. It must always be kept within a larger frame of reference. Businesses serve human persons not the other way around. As Pope John Paul says in *Centesimus Annus*:

> The Church acknowledges the legitimate role of profit as an indication that a business is functioning well. When a firm makes a profit, this means that productive factors have been properly employed and corresponding human needs have

---

129. *Centesimus Annus*, §§8, 17.

130. John Coverdale, "Why the Bottom Line Is not the Bottom Line: John Paul II's Concept of Business," *Journal of Catholic Legal Studies* 45, no. 2 (2006): 494. The model that dominates contemporary corporate legal scholarship is the "nexus of contracts" model of business which holds that corporations are nothing more than a nexus of contracts between a variety of stakeholders (shareholders, management, employees, clients, suppliers, etc.).

131. Martin, 10.

132. Coverdale, 494.

133. Coverdale.

134. Pope John Paul II, "Business Executives' Duty in an Age of Globalization," *The Pope Speaks*, 49, no. 5 (September-October 2004): 276.

been duly satisfied. But profitability is not the only indicator
of a firm's condition. It is possible for the financial accounts
to be in order, and yet for the people — who make up the
firm's most valuable asset — to be humiliated and their
dignity offended. Besides being morally inadmissible, this will
eventually have negative repercussions on the firm's economic
efficiency. In fact, the purpose of a business firm is not simply
to make a profit, but is to be found in its very existence as a
community of persons who in various ways are endeavoring
to satisfy their basic needs, and who form a particular group
at the service of the whole of society. Profit is a regulator of
the life of a business, but it is not the only one; other human
and moral factors must also be considered which, in the long
term, are at least equally important for the life of a business.[135]

What might such a business look like? Pope John Paul offers concrete
suggestions in *Laborem Exercens*, in which he calls us to see that:
(1) labor and capital cannot be opposed but are interdependent;
(2) moral economic systems recognize the priority of labor; and
(3) all recognize their dependence on the Creator. Again, he calls for a
way of envisioning the business enterprise as fundamentally rooted in
gift and always emphasizing the priority of persons over things (§13).
For example, as he notes:

> In the light of the above, the many proposals put
> forward by experts in Catholic social teaching and by
> the highest Magisterium of the Church take on special
> significance: *proposals for joint ownership of the means of
> work*, sharing by the workers in the management and/
> or profits of businesses, so-called shareholding by labor,
> etc. Whether these various proposals can or cannot be
> applied concretely, it is clear that recognition of the
> proper position of labor and the worker in the production

---

135. *Centesimus Annus*, §35. Here, profit refers simply to "revenues over expenses"; he does not here refer to profits-for-investors or owners.

process demands various adaptations in the sphere of the right to ownership of the means of production (§14).

Similarly, Pope Benedict calls for business practices that incorporate the principles of Catholic social doctrine, particularly the principle of gratuitousness. As many have noted, he proposes "hybrid forms of commercial enterprises":[136]

> Today we can say that economic life must be understood
> as a multi-layered phenomenon: in every one of these
> layers...the aspect of fraternal reciprocity must be present.
> In the global era, economic activity cannot prescind from
> gratuitousness, which fosters and disseminates solidarity
> and responsibility for justice and the common good among
> different economic players. It is clearly a specific and profound
> form of economic democracy. Solidarity is first and foremost a
> sense of responsibility on the part of everyone with regard to
> everyone, and it cannot therefore be merely delegated to the
> State. While in the past it was possible to argue that justice
> had to come first and gratuitousness could follow afterwards,
> as a complement, today it is clear that, without gratuitousness,
> there can be no justice in the first place. What is needed,
> therefore, is a market that permits the free operation, in
> conditions of equal opportunity, of enterprises in pursuit of
> different institutional ends. Alongside profit-oriented private
> enterprise and the various types of public enterprise, there
> must be room for commercial entities based on mutualist
> principles and pursuing social ends to take root and express
> themselves. It is from their reciprocal encounter in the

---

136. Michael Troilo provides an overview of hybrid enterprises in his excellent article "*Caritas in Veritate*, Hybrid Firms, and Institutional Arrangements," *Journal of Markets & Morality* 14, no. 1 (2011): 23-34. He identifies three types of hybrid enterprises: socially conscious firms (publically held firms that divert substantial resources to a social purpose but do pay shareholder dividends); socially oriented firms (privately held, divert a portion of the profit to retained earnings for future investment and a portion as a social dividend); and social output firms (offer a good or service to advance social welfare, e.g., low-cost dentistry). The latter do not return profits to shareholders but cannot pursue equity capital and must fund the enterprise from retained earnings (28-30).

marketplace that one may expect hybrid forms of commercial behavior to emerge, and hence an attentiveness to ways of *civilizing the economy*. Charity in truth, in this case, requires that shape and structure be given to those types of economic initiative which, without rejecting profit, aim at a higher goal than the mere logic of the exchange of equivalents, of profit as an end in itself (§38).

Specific phrases in these documents indicate key structural components of these hybrid institutions—joint ownership of the means of work, sharing by the workers in the management and/or profits of businesses, shareholding by labor, fraternal reciprocity, gratuitousness, economic democracy, mutualist principles, aim at a higher goal than profit as an end in itself.

A number of business models capture this vision of a hybrid institution. One example would be the Mondragón Corporation located in Spain. Founded in 1956 and structured explicitly according to the principles of Catholic social thought, it is currently the seventh largest company in Spain in terms of asset turnover. It is currently comprised of 258 companies, half of which are run as cooperatives, and which are divided into four areas—finance, industry, retail and knowledge. It employs over 83,000 people. It had over €14 billion in revenue in 2010, with €178 million of profit and €101 million of net investment. The organization is structured according to 10 basic principles that draw explicitly on Catholic social thought (see Appendix).[137]

Another business model, most likely underlying Pope Benedict's comments in *Caritas in Veritate*, is an organization known as the Economy of Communion (EOC).[138] Started in 1991 in Brazil by Chiara Lubich, who also founded the Catholic lay movement

---

137. David Herrera, "Mondragón: A For-Profit Organization that Embodies Catholic Social Thought," *Review of Business* 25, no. 1 (Winter 2004): 56-69. Also available at: http://www.stthomas.edu/cathstudies/cst/conferences/bilbao/papers/Herrera.pdf. For more information on the Mondragón Cooperativa, visit its website at: http://www.mondragon-corporation.com/ENG.aspx.

Focolare, the EOC is a worldwide network active in 182 countries, including the U.S., with about 100,000 adherents. It supports about 750 companies across business sectors. EOC businesses are committed to putting "people above profits" and to donating a portion of their profits to help the poor in developing nations or their local communities. They envision communion—between businesses and communities, between management and employees, between companies and recipients of aid—as the heart of economic life. They are very specific about how their profits are to be distributed: one third for direct aid for the poor, one third for educational support and formation that could help foster a culture of giving, and one third for the development of the businesses themselves.[139] They do not consider recipients of aid as "beneficiaries" but rather active participants in the project, people with whom they are in community and "communion."

Other examples of hybrid models embodying principles similar to that of Catholic social thought would be the Grameen Bank,[140] Muhammed Yunus' notion of the social business,[141] or the new

---

138. Jim Graves, "Radical Business Makeover: Rethinking the Balance of Profits and People Along Lines of Pope Benedict XVI's Social Encyclical," *Our Sunday Visitor* 99, no. 4 (May 23, 2010): 6. See also Amelia J. Uelmen, "*Caritas in Veritate*, and Chiara Lubich: Human Development from the Vantage Point of Unity," *Theological Studies* 71, no.1 (March 2010): 29-45.

139. Luigino Bruni & Amelia J. Uelmen, "What Is the Economy of Communion?" *Living City* 46 (June 2007): 12.

140. The Grameen Foundation: http://www.grameenfoundation.org. The Grameen Bank, initiative of Muhammad Yunus, was the pioneer microlending organization. Yunus and Grameen were awarded the Nobel Peace Prize in 2006. The bank lends primarily to poor women, making small loans ($25-$500), via a "solidarity-lending," community-support model. Grameen has evolved additional financial services based on this model, including a number of businesses and initiatives in the areas of health, communication technologies, agriculture and other fields. Grameen's philosophy is centered in an anthropology deeply resonant with that of the Catholic tradition. Borrowers are required to commit to a set of "Sixteen Decisions" which tie their financial progress to fundamental human and social goods. For example, they promise to repair their houses, maintain vegetable gardens for sustenance and sale, limit family size, educate their children, use latrines, live justly and so forth.

141. Yunus Social Business Global Initiatives: http://www.yunussb.com. Subsequent to the success of Grameen Bank, Muhammad Yunus developed the concept of social business, initially in partnership with Danone Corporation (makers of Dannon yogurt). Per its website, a social business is: "a non-dividend company created to solve a social problem. Like a non-governmental organization, it has a social mission, but, like a business, it generates its own revenues to cover its costs. *While investors may recoup their investment*, all further profits are reinvested into the same or other social businesses" (emphasis added).

innovation of "Benefit" or "B-Corps."[142] These are successful entrepreneurial economic endeavors that have very consciously and carefully structured principles akin to Catholic teaching into their corporate structures.[143] They consciously include such components as management by participatory democracy, strong commitments to donate a significant percentage of profits to community needs (job creation, education, care for the poor, etc.), the sharing of dividends/profits by all workers, limits on the differential between lowest and highest paid employees, and low and specific limits on dividends to investors/owners.

While all of these models, except for B-Corporations, were initially developed outside of the U.S., many now have U.S. affiliates.[144] Therefore, they all represent to some extent an attempt to embody the commitments of U.S. not-for-profit corporations—particularly significant community benefit—within a standard, capitalist economy. Importantly, however, beyond community benefit, they attend equally to the internal corporate relationships between management and labor, more authentically embodying the Catholic tradition's commitment to the priority of labor as a key manifestation of human dignity.

---

142. Benefit Corporation Information Center: http://benefitcorp.net. Benefit or B-Corps are a new type of for-profit corporation in the U.S. committed to a public, social good. The B-Corp movement was launched in 2010. Per its website: "Benefit Corporations are a new class of corporation that 1) creates a material positive impact on society and the environment; 2) expands fiduciary duty to require consideration of non-financial interests when making decisions; and 3) reports on its overall social and environmental performance using recognized third party standards." As for-profit, B-Corps return dividends to investors, but they are allowed to designate social goods that have a priority over profit and to specifically allocate a portion of their profits (e.g., 50 per cent) to that particular good. Some categorize them as "for-profit charities." B-Corp legislation has passed in about a dozen states and is pending in an additional 17.

143. Mohamad Yunus is Muslim, but there is a striking similarity between the principles that shape Grameen Bank, his vision of a social business, and the principles of Catholic social doctrine.

144. Mondragón began collaborating with U.S. Steel in 2009 (http://www.usw.org/media_center/releases_advisories?id=0234). Economy of Communion has U.S .affiliates as well.

5.4 CATHOLIC ECONOMIC THOUGHT AND CATHOLIC HEALTH CARE: THE FOR-PROFIT QUESTION

These primary commitments of Catholic social/economic thought and its vision of the business enterprise equip us to reflect more specifically on the question of corporate structures and Catholic health care. Echoing the popes' counsel, we might say that we find here a call *to develop profoundly new ways of understanding the enterprise of Catholic health care.*

This call applies not only to proposed for-profit possibilities but equally to the current not-for-profit structures of Catholic health care. Based on the foregoing commitments, we might ask: how do current not-for-profit health systems configure themselves in relation to the principles of Catholic economic thought? Do their corporate structures truly embody the vision of Catholic social and economic thought beyond charity care, particularly commitments to the dignity of labor, providing workers with a real voice in corporate decision making, the priority of labor over capital, small pay differentials between associates and senior leadership, and so on?[145] As many have noted, Catholic identity must encompass more than providing a specified amount of charity care and following the *Directives*.
In other words, the fundamental question is not only one of a simple distinction between for-profit or not-for-profit corporate structures, although the ends to which profits are directed remains an important issue. Rather what is required is a more thorough-going analysis of the ways in which the corporate structures of Catholic health care do or do not embody the central theological commitments of Catholic thought. The various examples offered in section 5.3 above—e.g., B-corporations, Mondragón, EOC, social businesses, socially conscious businesses—are offered here for three reasons. First, they are offered to stimulate the imagination. They are real-world examples of successful

---

145. One argument offered in favor of for-profit Catholic health care is that there is little difference in behavior between for-profit and not-for-profit Catholic health care institutions. While market pressures can certainly cause mission drift, the more appropriate conclusion from this premise is that not-for-profit institutions ought to start to behave more like not-for-profit institutions.

business ventures that can assist leaders in Catholic health care in thinking beyond the constraints imposed by business school curricula or our local contexts. How might such hybrid models be viable options for re-envisioning health care delivery in the new post-Accountable Care Act context, for either parent organizations or, perhaps on trial or pilot bases, for subsidiaries? Second, a number of these hybrid models are ventures founded by lay Catholics, seeking to lead faith-infused, economically successful business enterprises, and they have a long track-record of success in combining these goals. The standard U.S. not-for-profit model might not be the only way to combine real-world business with community benefit. Third, they remind us that as Catholics, we are members of a global church. The wisdom and experience embodied in these examples may lead to what's known as "reverse innovation"—the possibility that we in the U.S. could effectively learn from our global counterparts, particularly from their focus on human dignity, to adopt proven mechanisms that improve health outcomes and reduce costs.[146]

Certainly, contexts matter, particularly the larger context of health care delivery in the U.S. within which Catholic health care entities must function. As eminent Catholic health care ethicist Jack Glaser once observed: "a non-religious hospital in Germany has a far better chance of making biblical priorities present in German society than does a religious hospital in the United States. That is because the public policies shaping hospitals in Germany are significantly closer to biblical priorities than are similar parallel policies in this country."[147] Glaser makes this observation to call for Catholic health care to work toward systemic reform of the health care delivery system in the U.S. But it is also a call for Catholic health care to lead innovation—to creatively imagine new ways to embody biblical priorities, which can then serve as models for health care delivery more broadly.

---

146. M. Therese Lysaught, "Reverse Innovation from the Least of Our Neighbors," *Health Progress* 94, no. 1 (January-February 2013): 45-52.

147. Glaser and Glaser, 16.

We close this section by bringing the reflections in sections 5.1-5.3 to bear on the question of health care structures. Because the question of alternative corporate structures is relatively new, this section ends with more questions than conclusions. We pose hard questions designed to hone and sharpen the discernment process.

Integral human development, the priority of labor, and Catholic health care: Integral human development and the dignity/priority of labor are intertwined in this context. The claim is often made that the *structure* of a business does not matter as much as the end that it serves; that as long as a business serves a good end, the form of the business is irrelevant. However, as Catholic economic thought makes clear, structures embody assumptions, particularly assumptions about persons (are they simply "human resources" or "means of production"?). Structures also facilitate (or inhibit) movement toward certain ends: for example, requirements for tax-exempt not-for-profit organizations provide strong internal warrants and external pressures for prioritizing commitments to community benefit, especially when faced with tradeoffs.

Structures can also contribute to or undermine the integral development of persons. While "just treatment" of workers is important, Catholic social thought calls Catholic health care organizations to examine the ways in which their structures impact the integral development of associates. Arrangements such as joint ownership, participatory management and profit-sharing are not imperatives. But insofar as they embody a theologically grounded vision of the human person, new ways of envisioning participation and partnerships among various members of the health care organization as a "society of persons" or "community of solidarity" should be given serious consideration.[148]

---

148. As economist John Coverdale notes in his superb analysis of Pope John Paul's economic thought, "If we are to have an adequate legal framework for governing business, we cannot confine ourselves to questions about ownership and governance. We need to ask how we should structure business activity to reflect the proper role of work and economic activity in our personal and collective lives" (473-4). See Coverdale, "Why the Bottom Line Is Not the Bottom Line: John Paul II's Concept of Business," *Journal of Catholic Legal Studies* 45, no. 2 (2006) 473-521.

Structures of sin, solidarity and Catholic health care: Pope John Paul clearly correlates the "desire for profit" and the "idolatry of money" as one of the primary structures of sin. He repeatedly issues calls for the "priority of persons over profits." Pope Benedict repeats the call for new economic models and criticizes unregulated financial capitalism in his final address for the World Day of Peace.[149]

Such constant remarks throughout the literature provide an important reminder that the Catholic social tradition has always provided a both/ and approach in its economic analyses. While identifying strengths of capitalist economics, it has also always registered concerns and critiques. While Popes John Paul and Benedict call for new forms of business enterprise, there is as yet no evidence in the magisterial or theological literature that the church's affirmation of market economies, business or profit encompasses publicly traded, investor-owned or venture capital structures that function within the default assumptions of corporate law in the U.S. While the tradition does not reject these structures outright, the *theological* commitments provided by the Catholic economic tradition clearly point in a different direction. Thus, the bar for those who wish to justify standard U.S. investor-owned structures for Catholic health care over the variety of hybrid structures outlined above is high.

As one economist consulted for this paper noted, the hurdles separating Catholic identity and publicly traded, investor-owned or venture capital structures are, on a practical level, enormous. Certainly, it might be possible for such firms to satisfy the minimum conditions to be consistent with Catholic identity if they attempt to combine their for-profit structure with social goals. But are minimum conditions sufficient for the ministry of Catholic health care? New experiments in socially responsible businesses might bear fruit within Catholic health care, but firm conclusions regarding such a fit await long-term outcomes from these initiatives.

---

149. Benedict XVI, "Blessed Are the Peacemakers," Message for the World Day of Peace, January 1, 2013. Available at: http://www.vatican.va/holy_father/benedict_xvi/messages/peace/documents/hf_ben-xvi_mes_20121208_xlvi-world-day-peace_en.html.

Social goods and Catholic health care: Allied to the question of the corporate structure of health care delivery lies the larger unresolved question still debated within health care as a whole: is an investor-oriented for-profit structure for health care delivery appropriate *at all*, whether Catholic or not? This, of course, is not the simple question of paying for health care services. Paying for health care services does not necessarily mean commodifying health. Rather, the question is more complex. Is health care a social, public good, necessary not only for the good of each individual but for the common good as well? As early as 1995, Cardinal Bernardin argued precisely this point.[150] Catholic health care, by actively committing itself to the not-for-profit structure in the 1993 CHA discernment process as well as in CHA's constant advocacy for universal health care, answered in the affirmative. More recently, Sr. Gottemoeller observed:

> Health care is a necessary good, essential for human well-being. Hence, it cannot be treated as other goods that may be desirable but are not essential for human well-being. It is true that both for-profit and not-for-profit institutions vigorously compete for market share; can we say that each is equally motivated by a desire to improve the health of the community, with emphasis on the poor and underserved? I would suggest that a comparison of their community benefit expenditures might give the answer…Can [key characteristics of Catholic identity] be maintained and even optimized while discharging the required legal and fiduciary duties to bondholders and shareholders?[151]

---

150. Joseph Bernardin, "The Case for Not-for-Profit Health Care," *Origins* 24 (January 26, 1995): 538-42; Jean de Blois, "Can For-Profit Hospitals Be Catholic? No, Healthcare Is a Basic Human Right," *National Catholic Reporter* 34 (December 5, 2007): 20-1; Michael D. Place, "Agenda for the Strong at Heart: Facing the Challenges Ahead Will Require Recommitment to Our Right To Serve in a Manner Faithful to Our Identity," *Health Progress* 83, no. 4 (July-August 2002): 30-4, 58; and Edmund D. Pellegrino, "Ethical Issues in Managed Care: A Catholic Christian Perspective," *Christian Bioethics* 3, no. 1 (March 1, 1997): 55-73.

151. Gottemoeller, 2012, 34.

The papal tradition is very clear that fundamental human needs ought not be commodified and subject to market dynamics. Is health care one of those "human needs which find[s] no place in the market"? Is it, by justice, due to persons "by reason of [their] lofty dignity"? While the current not-for-profit structure of most of Catholic health care employs market mechanisms to deliver care, many rightly note that health care does not lend itself to the kind of market dynamics presumed by investor-owned models due a variety of factors, including the role of government funding and regulation as well as the nature of illness itself. Do investor-owned "mechanisms carry the risk of an 'idolatry' of the market, an idolatry which ignores the existence of goods which by their nature are not and cannot be mere commodities"?[152] This question of the nature of the good of health care, and the differences between health care and other industries, is a fundamental question to be answered during this discernment process.

Caritas and **Catholic health care:** Clearly, Catholic economic thought rejects any structure that makes the return of surplus revenue to investors or owners the *primary* end of the corporate enterprise. Returns to owners/investors must always be a subsidiary end, met only after the ends of patients/associates, communities and the organization itself. As noted above, it does appear that, per corporate law, *maximizing* shareholder or investor gain is only a default rule. As Macey notes, "shareholders could opt out of this goal if they so desired."[153] Therefore, in order to ameliorate the concern about shareholder primacy voiced by the range of stakeholders within Catholic health care, the articles of incorporation for corporate structures in Catholic health care would clearly need to specify the *primacy* of other goals as well as the specific ways that surplus revenues will serve those goals. Not-for-profit entities, by definition, already have a social good specified as their end or goal.[154] As we have seen, it is possible for alternative models of business enterprise

152. *Centesimus Annus*, §40.

153. Macey, 185.

154. Bernardin, 1995.

concretely to build *caritas* or the principle of gratuitousness into their articles of incorporation and business practices.

These principles of the Catholic social tradition, therefore, provide a compelling vision of the business enterprise and a framework for assessing potential corporate structures for Catholic health care. They move us beyond the simple question of for-profit or not-for-profit corporate structure to more carefully examine the ways in which various structures do or do not embody the central theological commitments of Catholic thought. What emerges is a range of possibilities by which Catholic health care, in its corporate embodiment, may advance the Kingdom of God by *civilizing the economy*, by understanding the organization as "a community of persons" which, "without rejecting profit, aim[s] at a higher goal than the mere logic of the exchange of equivalents, of profit as an end in itself." Which corporate forms, in other words, are structures embodying *caritas* in communion?

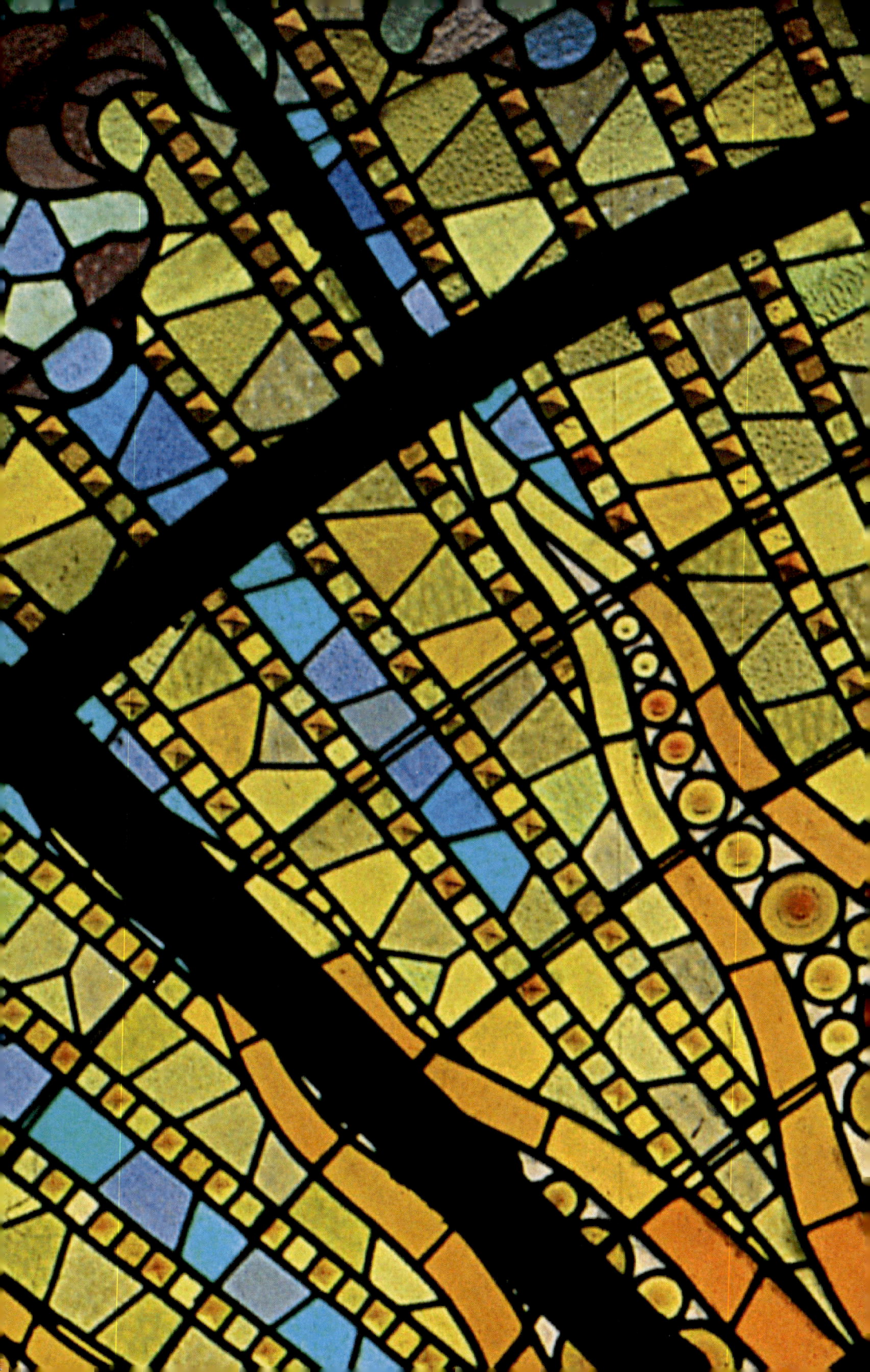

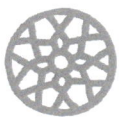

A S PROMISED, THE FOREGOING ANALYSIS OFFERS no recommendations regarding whether or how CHA should revise its membership criteria. Nor does it make specific suggestions regarding behaviors or markers of Catholic identity that health care institutions should adopt. It does not provide a checklist or a formula for assessing which health care institutions are Catholic. And it stakes no particular position on the for-profit versus not-for-profit question regarding Catholic health care.

The task of this study was to *identify the theological questions and analyses that might help inform CHA's discussions about membership.* More broadly, the task of this study was to identify the theological questions and fundamental commitments that ought to inform its discernment processes going forward. We hope that the study has achieved its purpose and will be of use to the Catholic health care ministry as it discerns not only around the adoption of various structures and partnerships, but as it discerns around new questions and issues that will undoubtedly emerge over the next few decades. Let us retrace our steps and name the theological questions identified here. We began with the notion of *identity* itself. We noted that the question of identity is always a question of looking backward and moving forward. It is a question of foundations and development in response to changing environments. The question of identity pushes us to assess the ways we change. Not all "change" is "progress." Taking time to reflect on the question of identity challenges us to ask: What is core, and why? What is essential, and why? How have we changed? Has that change been "progress"—development toward a worthy goal consistent with who we say we are? Or have circumstances in our context led us away from who we would like to be?

As we noted, this is fundamentally a question of *integrity*. Who *do* we say that we are? Why? On what grounds? Are our actions—including the ways we structure our lives and organizations—consistent with that identity? Will they move us toward a fuller embodiment of our identity, toward who we believe we are *called* to be? If so, how? How might particular actions or structures impede our ability to live our identity, to move toward our better selves?

If one studies the millennia-long history of Catholic health care and listens to the contemporary voices of those who carry on this important work today, certain theological warrants or groundings for *who we are* and *why we do what we do* emerge as central. None of these groundings stand alone. They form *a dynamic multi-faceted theological foundation*, the strength of which is reinforced by its multi-layered nature. The heart that shapes all these layers—the theological center of all that we are and do as Catholics—is *caritas*, God's love manifest in communion.

This communion-seeking *caritas* informs how we understand the other layers: the person and work of Jesus whose healing ministry we carry on; the person and work of the Spirit in the charisms of the founders of our hospitals and systems; the principles of Catholic social thought; our work as a ministry, a ministry that we share with the larger church; a ministry empowered by the grace of the sacraments; a ministry that entails witnessing to the faith through our embodied presence to our co-workers, our patients and our communities. This vision of the theological foundation of Catholic health care challenges us with hard questions: who do we understand Jesus to be? Do we see our work as a ministry? How do we understand the relationship between our organization and the church, both local and global?

Equally, practice often leads theory, and here the lived experience of Catholic health care identifies new theological issues that call for further study:

+ What are the Christologies (understandings of Jesus) that shape the work of various Catholic health care organizations?

+ How do we understand Catholic health care, theologically, as a ministry of the church—ministries led by lay people in non-ecclesial spaces, but necessarily in communion *as* church?

+ Might it be possible to develop an account of certain Catholic health care organizations as "works of Catholics" to accommodate their particularities (e.g., that not all within the ministry are Catholic, the nature of their partnerships, and so forth)?

+ How do we understand Catholic health care in light of the communion ecclesiology of Vatican II? How can/does/ought Catholic health care embody and participate in this ecclesiology in its most complete sense? How might it deepen that ecclesiology?

A theological foundation that at its heart seeks communion casts a new light on the principle of cooperation. We discovered in the tradition a broader context for understanding the principle. Pope Benedict affirms the positive theological mandate for Catholics to cooperate with others to advance the work of the Gospel and the development of persons and societies, to create communion. This mandate is based on a vision of God's love for each person which, through creation, sees all members of the human family as (ideally) one. Certainly questions of how to proceed in communion with others who are engaged in wrongdoing remains pressing, but this theological foundation for cooperation helps us to think about these more specific questions more accurately. Nonetheless, this analysis has identified a significant theological issue for further study:

+ What is a complete *theology* of cooperation and the principle of cooperation? What theological assumptions shaped the principle as it was developed, particularly in the 20TH century manuals? Are some of those theological assumptions at odds with the theological vision forwarded by Vatican II? If we are to use the principle of cooperation to analyze questions in 21ST century health care, in what ways will its theological assumptions need to be amended? How will that affect the ways the principle is interpreted and applied?

Our final question turned to that of structures. Which modes of such cooperative activity best enable the church—and particularly lay persons—to carry on the tradition of *caritas* in communion? In particular, can secular parent organizations, whether not-for-profit or for-profit, enable this work?

To address this question, we turned to economics. Here *caritas* in communion is translated, in the business context, into structures which embody these commitments along with the principle of gratuitousness and a particular vision of the business of Catholic health care as a community of persons. This vision not only raises questions about the fit between Catholic health care and particular for-profit structures; it poses equally hard challenges to current not-for-profit structures of Catholic health care.

Regarding both possibilities, the study concludes that there is no "no size fits all." As with many questions in the social tradition, the answer is not a simple "yes" or "no" but rather, *how?* As God's creation and the multiplicity of saints and religious orders attest, the incarnation of God's grace in the world is diverse and manifold. Grace transforms nature in ways that, most often, we cannot anticipate or imagine ahead of time; often, we do not recognize it when we see it.

At the same time, the witness of the Catholic tradition attests that when God's grace is incarnated in these manifold ways, it is often distinctive from the structures of business-as-usual in the world. It stands out as a new option, something thought not possible by conventional wisdom, something those who imagine the world without God will have a difficult time envisaging. But while distinctive, it will be clear that these manifold ways of embodying the Gospel (in this case, in Catholic health care) share something in common—though distinctive they will be connected to other institutions that claim the same identity.

As with the exploration of Catholic identity and cooperation, this study identified a number of areas requiring further research, particularly with regard to the actual experiences of Catholic hospitals and systems.

+ To what extent are Catholic hospitals/health systems now in partnerships with other-than-Catholic organizations?

+ To what extent have Catholic hospitals/health systems transitioned to for-profit corporate status and tried to maintain Catholic identity? What particular versions of "for-profit" structure have these transitions evolved?

+ To what extent do not-for-profit Catholic health systems have for-profit subsidiaries or have entered into joint ventures with for-profit entities? What models have been adopted in these instances? In which areas of health care have for-profit structures been adopted (e.g., revenue cycle, pharmacy, health plan, heart hospital, etc.)? What have been the outcomes relative to key components of Catholic identity in these subsidiaries?

To the extent possible, this research should expand beyond a simple qualitative study to be as quantitative and systematic as possible. It is anticipated that even with the year-long study proposed by CHA as phase-two of its discernment process, data will be ad hoc and sparse. An adequate assessment of these questions would require a study of multiple sites over a period of years.[155]

Additional background research and analysis would be helpful as well. A meta-analysis of studies comparing behavioral attributes and outcomes according to ownership structures (following the Thompson-Reuters 2010 study cited in footnote 156 below) would be of great assistance. The limited data set we have from Catholic for-profit hospitals and the broader data set comparing Catholic not-for-profit hospitals with for-profit and secular not-for-profit enterprises suggests that embodying Catholic identity is far more difficult for for-profit enterprises in the U.S. context than Catholic not-for-profit hospitals.[156]

A study of the track record of ethical accomplishments and lapses of for-profit health care companies would also be recommended. These studies would be particularly helpful in addressing the broader

---

155. We find in the literature a handful of articles defending the ability of for-profit Catholic hospitals to retain their Catholic identity, usually under the ownership of a secular, publically traded, for-profit parent entity. These articles, however, generally draw their conclusions from one example. In other words, they draw large conclusions from a very small data set. See Kelly Carroll, "Can For Profit Get the Mission Right?" *Health Progress* 93, no. 3 (May-June 2012): 49-59; Sheila Hammond, "Nurturing a Catholic Vision in a For-profit Hospital: Saint Louis University Hospital Fulfills a Promise To Carry Forward the Catholic Mission and Maintain Spiritual Care," *Health Progress* 90, no. 3 (May-June 2009): 57-9; James Clifton, "Can For-profit Hospitals Be Catholic? Yes, Hospital's Care of Indigent Has Grown," *National Catholic Reporter* 34 (December 5, 1997): 20-1. Clifton tells the story of St. Joseph Mercy Hospital in Omaha that, due to its inability to maintain Catholic identity under for-profit ownership, separated from Tenet Healthcare Corporation in 2013. CHA should make sure that its conclusions from Year Two of the discernment process are well supported by data.

question of whether health care, per se, and the well-being of associates and patients, is advanced or diminished under for-profit corporate structures.

A final set of questions emerges from the interface of theology and practice. Bringing Parts III and V into conversation, questions that remain unanswered within the Catholic social tradition would include:

+ Are for-profit corporate structures legitimate for ministries of the church? If so, are some versions of for-profit structures more fitting than others? Ought *ministries* be held to a different standard of economic practice than secular business enterprises? Why or why not?

+ Are for-profit corporate structures legitimate ways to embody a sacramental Catholic work, such as continuing the healing mission of Jesus?

We have, then, a rich agenda for further research, and a rich resource here to guide future discernment. This discernment will be a great resource for the church and theological wisdom, informing theology with practice. Yet, while practice often leads theory/theology, theology also necessarily guides practice, ensuring integrity, keeping lived experience faithful to its identity, joining those who share a common identity in union and communion.

---

156. Studies suggest that Catholic health systems, in their current not-for-profit form, demonstrate greater quality and efficiency than other for-profit or investor owned systems, as well as more compassionate care services (palliative care, HIV/AIDS, behavioral health). Not-for-profit systems demonstrate lower mortality rates, lower price markup, "are more likely to provide health promotion services, support safety-net providers, collaborate to meet community needs, conduct community health assessments and work with local health departments," and foster more innovation. David Foster, *Differences in Health System Quality Performance by Ownership*, Thomson-Reuters, August 9, 2010 (available at: http://www.100tophospitals.com/assets/100TOPSystemOwnership.pdf). "Catholic Health Care Rated High," *National Catholic Reporter*, August 20, 2010, 3; Carroll, 51; Clarke E. Cochran and Kenneth R. White, "Does Catholic Sponsorship Matter?" *Health Progress 83*, no. 1 (January-February 2002): 15. In 2007, Catholic health systems reported $5.7 billion in community benefit. How does the community benefit track record of for-profit health systems in the U.S. compare? See CHA Community Benefit website, "May 2007 National Reporting Campaign." http://www.chausa.org/Pages/Our_Work/Community_Benefit/Ministry_Examples/May_2007_National_Reporting_Campaign/Overview/.

We hope that this study, in conjunction with the continuing discernment facilitated by CHA as well as theologians and Catholic scholars, will enable Catholic health systems and hospitals, empowered by the principle of subsidiarity, to determine which models of corporate structure and partnership best embody their identity with integrity in the particular communities in which they are located. We also hope that this study enables the ministry as a whole to discern together around its experience, the market realities of contemporary health care, and its commitment to Catholic identity as it continues to lead the church and the world in envisaging new forms of engagement, commitment, cooperation and, now, new ways of understanding the health care enterprise that advance the healing mission of Jesus Christ in the world for the common good and the good of the Kingdom.

QUESTIONS FOR REFLECTION AND DISCUSSION

1. Faithfulness to Catholic identity demands the question of integrity—who we say we are and what we believe we are called to be. How might particular actions or structures impede our ability to live our identity with integrity?

2. How might particular actions or structures support and enhance the ability of Catholic health care to live out the ministry of Jesus?

3. What are some real experiences of Catholic health care ministries that have sought to create new collaborative structures? Which raise cautionary concerns? Which give hope for new ways to advance the healing mission of Jesus?

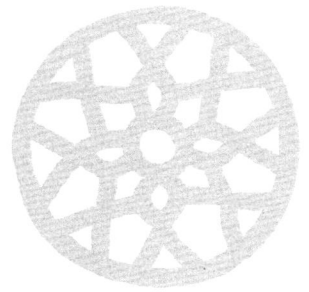

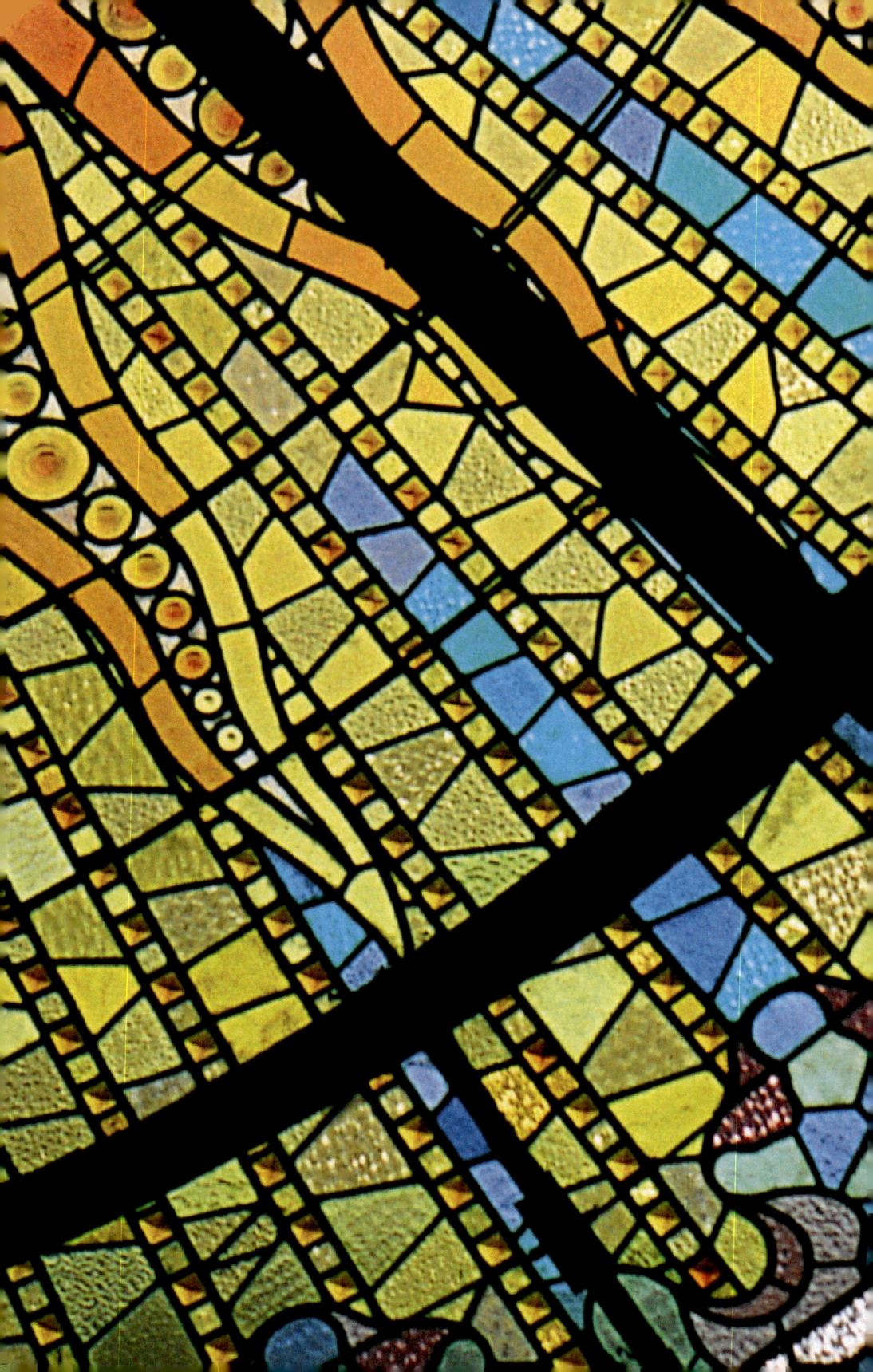

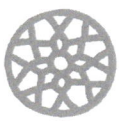

APPENDIX

TEN BASIC PRINCIPLES OF MONDRAGÓN

(ORMAECHEA, J. M., 1993)

(FROM DAVID HERRERA)

THE MONDRAGÓN ORGANIZATION IS GROUNDED on 10 basic principles that balance individual, organizational and community needs:

Open admission. Mondragón is open to all persons who are capable of carrying out the available jobs. There is no discrimination based on religious or political grounds, nor due to race, gender, age or socio-economic levels. The only requirement is the acceptance of these Basic Principles.

Democratic organization. Workers are owners, and owners are workers. Each cooperative is managed by a system of "one person-one vote."

Sovereignty of employee's work over capital. Workers join Mondragón and become owners after making a capital contribution at the end of a trial period. All workers are entitled to an equitable distribution of profits. The return on saved or invested capital is just but limited and it is not tied up to the surpluses or losses of the cooperatives.

Subordinate character of capital. Capital is a means to an end, not an end in itself. Available capital is used primarily to create more jobs.

Participatory management. Worker-owners participate in decision making and the management of the cooperatives. This implies development of self-management skills. Formal education and adequate information is provided to improve worker-owners' ability to participate competently in decision making.

Payment solidarity. Remuneration is regulated internally and externally. Internally, an agreed differential between the highest and lowest paid job is applied. Externally, a remuneration level is maintained in relationship with similar local industries.

Intercooperation. Cooperatives form Groups to pool profits, to absorb worker-owner transfers when necessary, and to attain synergies. These Groups associate with each other to support corporate institutions. Mondragón associates with other Basque cooperative organizations to promote the cooperative model.

Social transformation. Mondragón cooperatives invest a majority of their profits in the creation of new jobs. Funds are also used in community projects and in institutions that promote the Basque culture and language.

Universal nature. Mondragón proclaims its solidarity with other cooperative movements, with those working for economic democracy and with those who champion the objectives of peace, justice and human dignity. Mondragón proclaims its solidarity especially with people in developing countries.

Education. Mondragón cooperatives commit the required human and economic resources to basic, professional and cooperative education in order to have worker-owners capable of applying all basic principles mentioned above.

Caritas in Communion: A Summary

BY KAREN SUE SMITH

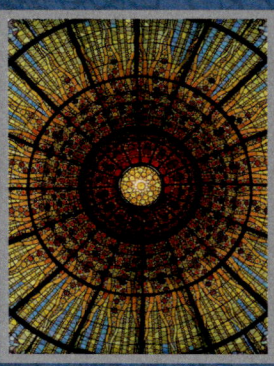

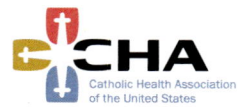

Catholic Health Association of the United States
A Passionate Voice for Compassionate Care

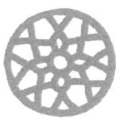

CARITAS IN COMMUNION: A SUMMARY

ATHOLIC HEALTH CARE FINDS ITSELF WITHIN A
rapidly changing landscape. In response, some Catholic
hospitals and collaborative health systems are making
structural changes. Some systems have decided to forgo
formal recognition by their diocesan bishops, for example, while a
few hospitals and systems have begun to explore for-profit corporate
structures. These and other new models-in-the-making may have
deep, far reaching implications for their ministries, implications still
unknown. Meanwhile, the self-identity of many of these institutions
is changing. Mixed models of identity have emerged, models no
longer solely Catholic but with ecumenical, interfaith or secular
dimensions. Mixed models of identity intensify such basic questions
as: What makes Catholic health care *Catholic*? Can an organization
maintain its Catholic identity if it is owned and/or managed by an
other-than-Catholic organization? If so, how? How might for-profit
status affect Catholic identity?

For CHA, these new developments also raise a practical issue.
Currently, the association's criteria for membership require both "not-
for-profit" status and recognition as Catholic by the diocesan bishop.
Given this disconnect, the CHA Board of Trustees has outlined

a three-year discernment process to help members reflect on the theological foundations of Catholic health care (year one), consider in light of those foundations the experience of members that have adopted new models (year two), and revisit the CHA membership criteria (year three).

"*Caritas* in Communion," the study upon which this summary is based, is a fruit of year one. Written with wide consultation, it accounts for the theological commitments that ground Catholic health care ministry. Specifically, the study examines the theological foundations of three pivotal issues: **Catholic identity** in Catholic health care, the **principle of moral cooperation** used to assess partnerships between Catholic and other institutions, and Catholic economic thought as it pertains to **for-profit status** in health care.

In framing and analyzing how the new models relate to traditional Catholic health care organizations, a series of questions may prove helpful. What is the religious identity of the parent organization? of individual hospitals? What is the for-profit/not-for-profit status of each? How are the relationships between Catholic and other-than-Catholic components of the system structured? What is the relationship between the system, hospitals and diocesan bishops? What is the role of the sponsors?

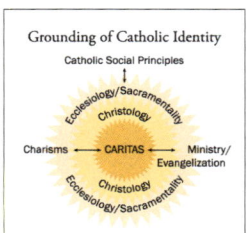

1. CATHOLIC IDENTITY

Catholic health care organizations are envisioning new ways to maintain their Catholic identity within new structures. They are taking steps to remain in relationship with the diocesan bishop and the sponsors. They continue to follow the *Ethical and Religious Directives for Catholic Health Care Services*, to offer pastoral care and the sacraments and to provide charity care. Are all of these vital to Catholic identity? Are they sufficient?

Catholic identity is a complex term. Its meaning has been debated since the 1970s. "Identity" itself has many dimensions. It concerns intrinsic characteristics of a person or institution that are consistent over time, are perceivable by others, distinguish a person or institution and connect them to others. Yet identity also develops over time in response to experience. All persons and institutions embody multiple identities simultaneously. Discerning the core characteristics of one's identity is an ongoing process attuned to place and time. *Catholic* identity is embedded in Catholic tradition, which includes spirituality and prayer, the church's sacramental and liturgical life and official church teaching. While Catholic identity is neither fixed nor complete, it does have roots. And it should be perceptible to others. We ask *who do we say we are?* in order to discern who we are called to be, and what we ought to do in new situations.

Consensus is emerging around seven characteristics of Catholic identity in health care. Catholic health care is rooted in and continues to make present in the world: (1) the healing ministry of Jesus, (2) the stories of the founding congregations and (3) the social teaching of the church. Catholic health care is also (4) a ministry of the church, (5) a sacrament or sign of Christ's presence, (6) a way of being in communion with the church and (7) a means of witnessing to the faith.

Beneath the key characteristics we find several theological concepts that ground Catholic identity. Catholic health care draws its identity, for example, from a balanced Christology based on Jesus' dual nature as both human and divine. The results are practical. In continuing the healing ministry of Jesus, Catholic health care tends to body and spirit, to the welfare of patients and their families, as well as to staff/employees. Similarly, the stories of the founding congregations not only inspire us, but invite us to share their charism and close links to Jesus, bringing that grace and power into the present. The church's social teaching—with its emphasis on human dignity, the common good, stewardship, solidarity, subsidiarity, care for the whole person, concern for the poor and vulnerable—also is made present, affirmed in the *Directives,* in employee compensation and benefits, in charity care and other ways.

Catholic health care recognizes itself as a ministry, though historically the word "ministry" has been limited to the work of the clergy. The Second Vatican Council's Dogmatic Constitution on the Church (*Lumen Gentium*), however, shifted the sacramental basis of Christian work in the world from ordination to baptism. Since then, theology has begun to describe the work of the laity, grounded in baptism, as ministry. This theology is still evolving. So far, neither lay ecclesial ministry (modeled on parish life) nor the works of religious institutes is an exact fit for Catholic health care.

Ecclesiology (the theology of the church) also is evolving in its understanding of church as communion. The "communion ecclesiology" of Vatican II presents the church as founded in baptism and created anew each time the Eucharist is celebrated. The people of God who make up the church share the "priesthood of the faithful." Historically, for Catholic health care to be in communion meant to have validation from the diocesan bishop. Today that seems insufficient as health care systems now extend beyond diocesan borders; the link with the church needs clarification. In the 1970s, Catholic health care developed the role of sponsor and appropriated the canonical "public juridic person" in an effort to maintain an official connection between religious institutes, their lay-led ministries and the church. Sponsorship continues to move Catholic health care toward a more complete understanding of communion ecclesiology, a fuller vision of the shared work of laity, vowed religious and bishops.

Jesus commissioned the church to be the visible sign (or sacrament) of God's salvation. Thus sacramentality is central to Catholic health care. Catholic institutions not only continue to provide the sacraments to patients and staff, they perform their daily work as a visible sign of Christ in the world. Those who work in Catholic health care are called to embody Christ as healer. This sacramentality includes ordinary moments, like serving hospital food, wiping the drool from the chin of an Alzheimer's patient, covering a naked patient, and other daily encounters—occasions of grace.

Witnessing to the faith is reflected in the way Catholic institutions treat persons of all faiths or no faith. To witness does not mean to proselytize, even though some patients and staff, influenced by the lives of nurses and other practitioners, have converted or become reconciled to God. Witness is the way Catholic health care, by continuing God's healing work, invites people to God.

These seven characteristics of Catholic identity are interrelated in layers around *caritas* ("*love*" or "*charity*" in some translations). *Caritas* is the theological reality upon which the cosmos is created and sustained, thus the bedrock on which Catholic health care stands. Pope Benedict's encyclicals "God Is Love" (*Deus Caritas Est*) and "Charity in Truth" (*Caritas in Veritate*) describe *caritas*, a concept that far exceeds the notion of "charity care." *Caritas* is the very essence of God. It is the way God interacts with the world. *Caritas* is essential to all that derives from God. It follows that *caritas* is the essence of the person Jesus Christ; the essence of the church; the essence of the sacraments by which we encounter God; the essence of ministry; the essence of witness; the essence of Catholic social principles; and the essence of the stories of the founders of Catholic health care.

Catholic health care is a concrete practice of love. It takes shape as a communion of people engaged in ministry and witness, steeped in Catholic social thought and the Spirit-led charisms of our founders, which continue to inspire our ministry. Catholic health care is sacramental, grounded in an ecclesiology rooted in Christ, the summit and fullness of God's *caritas* in the world.

2. THE PRINCIPLE OF MORAL COOPERATION

Catholic health care tries to demonstrate *caritas*, showing what health care looks like when shaped by a community witnessing to God's love. Yet Catholic identity has been difficult to maintain within the traditional models. How might emerging models further complicate the challenges?

To date, the ethical principle of moral cooperation has been a primary lens used to assess the implications of partnerships between Catholic and other-than-Catholic organizations. The principle enables us to determine what involvements with others are morally acceptable. It suggests what to do when one discovers that the good one does involves one in some wrongdoing of another. Yet as used in Catholic health care today the principle has limitations. For one thing, the principle was developed in the 16th century to help priests hear confessions, assess sins and assign penances, leading a penitent to reconciliation. Since the 1990s moral theologians have debated whether the principle is applicable to institutions like health care. Also, the principle does not reflect the robust ecclesiology emerging from Vatican II in which the church, seeing itself as a part of the modern world, is obliged to engage with it. A more fully developed "theology of cooperation" on which to ground the principle may help Catholic health systems determine how to advance the Kingdom through other-than-Catholic structures.

The writings of Popes Paul, John Paul, and Benedict have begun to articulate such a theology. The church has recognized that Christians have a positive obligation to cooperate with others, including the State, and those of other faiths. In "Charity in Truth" Pope Benedict states the basis for collaboration, describing the human race as "a single family working together in true communion." Joint efforts with others must be mutual and transparent, Pope Benedict writes. And partners in collaboration must be open to faith that is "purified by reason" and reason "purified by faith." The purpose of collaboration is to further justice, peace and human development.

Pope Benedict identifies the primary theological grounding for the mandate to collaborate as the doctrine of charity (*caritas*). He finds additional grounds for collaboration in theological anthropology, ministry and evangelization, the church's social teaching and the goodness of creation. Pope Benedict's theology reveals a positive understanding of the relationship between church and world. Moreover, laypersons are to be the primary agents of this collaboration. In 2012, Pope Benedict forcefully said that laypersons should "not be regarded as 'collaborators' of the clergy but rather as people who are really 'co-responsible' for the church's being and acting."

The principle of cooperation and assessments about Catholic partnerships, then, must be interpreted and applied within a rich theology of cooperation. That theology has roots in the unity of the human family and in the doctrine of *caritas*. It reflects a positive vision of relations between church and world and an increasing appreciation of the co-responsibility of the laity for the church.

In light of current papal theology, then, Catholic health care finds itself not only permitted to enter into partnerships with other faith-based and secular organizations; it finds a positive obligation to engage in "*fraternal collaboration between believers and non-believers*" ("Charity and Truth"). Consider that throughout the world access to affordable care is an issue of justice and peace. Often the health needs of the public are more effectively served by collaborative efforts. In Catholic health care these efforts are typically lay-led. Collaboration between Catholics and other-than-Catholics bears fruit for the Gospel and human development in society. Catholic systems in partnership not only deliver health care across populations, especially to the poor and marginalized, but have been remarkably successful in influencing other institutions to adopt many Catholic values. Their success in achieving *practical* moral consensus is unparalleled in the United States.

This theological analysis calls for a new approach to the principle of cooperation, one that moves discussions away from a narrow focus (on reproductive issues, for example) toward the overall mission of Catholic health care. Conversation would build on the goods we hold in common. It would follow the church's approach to the collaboration of institutions in the social sphere, rather than of individuals in the personal sphere. And it would align the principle of cooperation with Catholic social thought regarding the promotion of the common good and the proper subsidiarity of other-than-Catholic partners.

If other-than-Catholic (secular) not-for-profit parent organizations are structured to allow all participants their proper subsidiarity, they may prove amenable to the maintenance of Catholic identity within hospitals and subsystems. They may even allow for a greater range of Catholic partnerships with other faith-based or secular providers of health care, increasing the scope of the work of charity in the world.

The main question regarding new partnerships is: Does the structure of a proposed organization—especially where one party is managed by the other—diminish/preserve/enhance the mutuality necessary for dialogue and true collaboration?

3. THE FOR-PROFIT QUESTION

Since there is no authoritative doctrinal teaching on the question of whether Catholic ministries ought to adopt for-profit or not-for-profit corporate status, this study outlines the theological parameters for discernment. The goal is to shed theological light on the question: Is a shift to for-profit status for an organization in Catholic health care consistent with Catholic identity? To do so, we look at magisterial teaching on economics, applicable social questions and the theology behind them.

First, two definitions. **A for-profit corporation** (whether publicly traded or privately held) is one that intends to maximize the shareholder value, which can include returning a portion of surplus revenues to owners or investors. **A not-for-profit corporation** cannot distribute surplus revenues as profits or dividends to owners or investors, but rather must use surplus revenues to achieve other specified goals; these goals include preserving or expanding the corporation itself or funding community goods.

The main concern about shifting to for-profit status in Catholic health care is "shareholder primacy." Shareholder primacy holds that corporations are obligated to make profit-for-owners the primary end to which all other ends are secondary. A strong cultural assumption, taught in business schools and upheld in case law, is that for-profit corporations are obliged to maximize profits for shareholders. Still, as some have argued, pursuit of humanitarian, charitable, social or other stakeholder objectives is legally within the discretion of for-profit corporate leadership.

Catholic social doctrine speaks of the economy in particular terms. It speaks of integral human development, the dignity and priority of labor, structures of sin and solidarity, private property and the universal destination of goods and the principle of gratuitousness. All five principles bear on our question.

+ *Integral human development* places corporate profits in subordination to other goods, such as the full flourishing of the common good. As John Paul II writes in "On Human Work," integral human development through work "does not impede but rather promotes the greater productivity and efficiency of work itself."

+ Regarding *human labor*, Pope John Paul affirms the priority of labor over capital, of persons over profit. The reason is that work is more than wages. Work is the primary activity by which persons move toward their fulfillment and advance toward human flourishing.

+ As for *structures of sin*, Pope John Paul urges the citizens of rich countries to examine their relationship to world poverty. He points to the "all-consuming desire for profit" as an example of structural sin that misdirects economies in ways that cause or perpetuate poverty. The antidote is solidarity with others and a commitment to the common good.

+ Catholic teaching, since Pope Leo, has upheld the right to *private property*. But Pope John Paul also notes limitations on the right, which concern the *universal destination of goods*. Since the goods of creation are given by God for all, the right to private property is always qualified by the basic needs of others for material survival and the good of the community.

+ In "Charity in Truth," Pope Benedict adds the *principle of gratuitousness* to Catholic economic thought. Since God's presence and all the goods of creation are freely given to the world, then "economic, social and political development...needs to make room for the principle of gratuitousness as an expression of fraternity." Pope Benedict challenges the marketplace, especially Catholic institutions, to create space "for economic activity to be carried out by subjects who freely choose to act according to principles other than those of pure profit, without sacrificing the production of economic value in the process. The many economic entities that draw their origin from religious and lay initiatives demonstrate that this is concretely possible." The powerful economic reality of Catholic health care was (and still is) made possible by the logic of gift.

Whereas in *unbridled capitalism* the human person may be reduced to an instrument of production, in Catholic thought capitalism is *always bridled* by the dignity of the human person and the common good of society. Pope John Paul urges Christians to pursue profit "with a deeper concern for the spread of solidarity and the elimination of the scourge of poverty." Profit cannot be the sole or even primary factor directing corporate life. Instead, Pope John Paul sees labor and capital as interdependent—a business can be jointly owned, its profits shared with workers, its corporate decisions made with worker input. Pope Benedict proposes the creation of "hybrid forms of commercial enterprises." If the economy is to be "civilized," to aim at a higher goal than mere profit, he writes, there must be room for "commercial entities based on mutualist principles and pursuing social ends to take root and express themselves."

Consider four real-world examples of alternative corporations that put people above profits: the Mondragón Corporation, a major employer in Spain; the Economy of Communion, a worldwide organization begun in Brazil by Chiara Lubich, founder of Focolare; the Grameen Bank, a microlender, founded in Bangladesh by Muhammed Yunus; and the "Benefit" corporations or "B-Corps," which seek to influence society and the environment positively in addition to making a profit. These hybrids embody commitments like those of U.S. not-for-profit corporations, particularly community benefit.

Catholic social thought calls us to develop profoundly new ways of understanding the enterprise of Catholic health care. The challenge applies to both not-for-profit corporations and those with for-profit structural elements. Do our corporate structures embody the vision of Catholic social and economic thought beyond charity care, particularly commitments to the dignity of labor, giving workers a real voice in corporate decision making, the priority of labor over capital, small pay differentials between associates and senior leadership? As a global church, we in the United States can learn much from imaginative examples beyond our borders. Catholic health in the U.S. could become a leader in innovation, modeling biblical priorities in health care delivery. How might hybrid models be made viable for either parent organizations or subsidiaries as we re-envision health care this post-Affordable Care Act period?

To sharpen the discernment process, we identify the following points:

+ Structures matter. Business structures embody assumptions about persons and economic goals—integral human development and the priority of labor, for example. Structures can and should be devised to reflect a theologically grounded vision.

+ Catholic social tradition provides a both/and approach to economic analysis; it notes the strengths and weaknesses of market economies. While the church does not reject publicly traded, investor-owned or venture capital structures, its theological commitments point in a direction other than maximizing profits for shareholders. For that reason, the bar must be set high when it comes to choosing standard U.S. investor-owned structures for health care over not-for-profit or hybrid structures.

+ A prior question about health care as a fundamental good deserves consideration. Papal teaching makes clear that basic human needs ought not be commodified and subject to market dynamics. Is health care one of those "human needs"? If so, does it lend itself to investor-owned models?

+ Catholic economic thought, built on the doctrine of *caritas*, rejects any structure that makes shareholder profits the primary goal. Maximizing shareholder profits is a default rule, however, that shareholders can reject. The articles of incorporation for Catholic health care can specify the primacy of some other goal, as well as the specific ways that surplus revenues will serve those goals. Alternative models can build *caritas* or the principle of gratuitousness into their articles of incorporation and business practice.

This analysis leads us to examine the ways in which various structures do or do not embody the central theological commitments of Catholic thought. For Catholic health care can advance God's Kingdom in many ways, including civilizing the economy by placing the good of the human community as a higher goal than profit. The foundational question is: Which corporate structures, including new hybrids (some yet to be imagined), best enable the embodiment of the tradition of *caritas* in communion? In answering this question, the issue of Catholic identity will find resolution.

QUESTIONS FOR REFLECTION AND DISCUSSION

CATHOLIC IDENTITY

Catholic identity, *who we say we are,* should be perceptible to others.

+ In what visible ways does your system/facility make its Catholic identity "perceptible to others"?

+ How is Catholic identity perceptible in *the way people relate to one another* in your system/facility?

PRINCIPLE OF MORAL COOPERATION

Pope Benedict said that laypersons should be "regarded as people who are really 'co-responsible' for the church's being and acting."

+ In your system/facility is there a spirit of "co-responsibility" for the ministry?

+ How is it expressed by executive leadership?

+ How is it expressed by all associates?

+ Is it felt and experienced by those who receive care?

+ In considering and negotiating a new relationship and structure
  with another entity, through what process would you incorporate a
  spirit of co-responsibility? With an other-than-Catholic entity? With
  a for-profit entity?

THE FOR-PROFIT QUESTION

Within the context of Catholic social doctrine, Pope John Paul
affirmed the priority of labor over capital and of persons over profit
and that "work is the primary activity by which persons move toward
their fulfillment and advance toward human flourishing."

+ How would you address negotiations regarding the work force for a
  Catholic system/facility that is considering entering into partnership
  with a for-profit entity?

+ As a leader in the process, how do you integrate the concepts of *the
  dignity of the human person* and *the common good of society* into the
  decision making process?

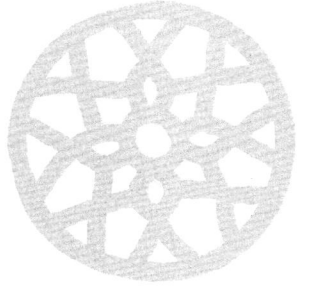

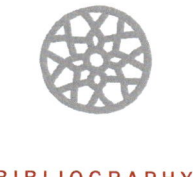

BIBLIOGRAPHY

CATHOLIC IDENTITY

"Hospitals Enter Debate Over Catholic Identity." *National Catholic Reporter* 34 (November 7, 1997): 20.

"Maintaining Catholic Identity." *Health Progress* 80, no. 4 (July-August 1999): 41-3.

Arbuckle, Gerald. *Healthcare Ministry: Refounding the Mission in Turbulent Times.* Collegeville, Minn.: Liturgical Press, 2000.

Bancroft, Nancy Parent. "The 'Next Generation' Model." *Health Progress* 85, no. 3 (May-June 2004): 27-30, 55.

Benedict XVI. "The Co-Responsibility of the Laity." *Origins* 42, no. 16 (September 20, 2012): 254-5.

Bernardin, Joseph L. "Catholic Institutions and Their Identity." *Origins* 21, no. 2 (May 23, 1991): 33-6.

Bevans, Stephen B. *An Introduction to Theology in Global Perspective.* Maryknoll, N.Y.: Orbis, 2009.

Bisson, Diane. "Institutional Integrity: Values in Action." *Health Progress* 83, no. 2 (March-April 2002): 10-12, 52.

Bouchard, Charles E. "Health Care as 'Ministry': Common Usage, Confused Theology." *Health Progress* 89, no. 3 (May-June 2008): 26-30.

_____. "The Four Ages: We've Only Just Begun." *Health Progress* 82, no. 5 (September-October 2001): 9, 82.

_____. "Catholic Healthcare and the Common Good." *Health Progress* 80, no. 3 (May-June 1999): 34-40.

Boyle, Joseph. "Catholic Health Care Institutions and Modern Health Care Delivery." *Christian Bioethics* 5, no. 1 (1999): 3-4.

Bradel, William T., Virginia Gillis, Jim Harkness, Terrance P. McGuire, and Tom Nehring. "Integrating Cultures." *Health Progress* 80, no. 2 (March-April 1999): 65-78.

Brady, Jane Frances. "Charism and Identity: Signs of Hope in Catholic Health Care." *Hospital Progress* 63, no. 11 (November 1982): 38-41.

Brinkmann, Bill., T. Dean Maines, Michael J. Naughton, J. Michael Stebbins, and Arnold Weimerskirch. "Bridging the Gap. Catholic Health Care Organizations Need Concrete Ways to Connect Social Principles to Practice." *Health Progress* 87, no. 6 (November-December 2006): 43-50.

Buckley, Michael J. *The Catholic University as Promise and Project: Reflections in a Jesuit Idiom.* Washington, D.C.: Georgetown University Press, 1999.

Burnside, Gordon. "A Ministry of Presence." *Health Progress* 82, no. 6 (November-December 2001): 52, 55, 78.

Butler, Francis J. *American Catholic Identity: Essays in an Age of Change.* Kansas City, Mo: Sheed & Ward, 1994.

Cacciavillan, Agostino. "Catholic Identity: Both Love and Truth Are Essential." *Origins* 28, no. 24 (November 26, 1998): 421-3.

Cafardi, Nicholas P., and Adam J. Maida. "Charitable Trust Helps Ensure Catholic Hospitals' Identity." *Hospital Progress* 63, no. 9 (September 1982): 32-5.

Casey, Juliana. "Holy Memory, Faithful Action." *Health Progress* 81, no. 2 (March-April 2000): 28-31.

_____. *Food for the Journey: Theological Foundations for Catholic Health Care.* St. Louis, Mo: Catholic Health Association, 1991.

Cassidy, Judy. "Catholic Identity Is Based on Flexible, Reasonable Tradition." *Health Progress* 75, no. 1 (January-February 1994): 16, 25.

Catholic Bishops of New Jersey. "The Rationale of Catholic Health Care." *Origins* 25, no. 27 (December 21, 1995): 449, 451-2.

Catholic Health Association. "How To Approach Catholic Identity in Changing Times." *Health Progress* 75, no. 5 (May 1994): 23-9.

Catholic Health Association. *Toward a Theology of Catholic Health Care Sponsorship.* St. Louis, Mo: Catholic Health Association, 2005.

Chapp, Larry S. "Negotiating Identity: Catholic Higher Education Since 1960." *Thomist* 65, no. 3 (July 2001): 481-4.

Chaput, Charles. "The Future of the Catholic Health Care Vocation." *Origins* 39, no. 40 (March 18, 2010): 654-8.

Christiansen, Drew. "Measuring Catholic Identity." *America* 194, no. 11 (March 27, 2006): 5.

Clifford, Anne M. "Identity and Vision at Catholic Colleges and Universities." *Horizons* 35, no. 2 (Fall 2008): 355-70.

Cochran, Clarke E. "Catholic Healthcare in the Public Square: Tension on the Frontier." In *Handbook of Bioethics and Religion*, edited by David Guinn. New York, N.Y.: Oxford University Press, 2006.

_____. "Renewing the Sacramental." *Health Progress* 84, no. 6 (November-December 2003): 12-5.

_____ and Kenneth R. White. "Does Catholic Sponsorship Matter?" *Health Progress* 83, no. 1 (January-February 2002): 14.

_____. "Another Identity Crisis: Catholic Hospitals Face Hard Choices." *Commonweal* 127, no. 4 (February 25, 2000): 12-6.

_____. "Institutional Identity, Sacramental Potential: Catholic Healthcare at Century's End." *Christian Bioethics* 5, no. 1 (1999): 26-43.

_____. "Sacrament and Solidarity: Catholic Social Thought and Healthcare Policy Reform." *Journal of Church and State* 41, no. 3 (Summer 1999): 475-498.

Coleman, John A. "Catholic Identity." *America* 182, no. 16 (May 6, 2000): 18-20.

Connelly, Michael D. "Together We Can Do More." *Health Progress* 80, no. 4 (July-August 1999): 80.

Cox, William J. "Nurturing the Ministry's Soul." *Health Progress* 85, no. 5 (September-October 2004): 38-43.

Curley, John E., Jr. "Catholic Identity, Catholic Integrity." *Health Progress* 72, no. 8 (October 1991): 56-60.

Curran, Charles E. "The Catholic Identity of Catholic Institutions." *Theological Studies* 58, no. 1 (March 1997): 90-108.

Cusack, Barbara Anne. "The Role of the Diocesan Bishop in Relation to Catholic Health Care." *Health Progress* 87, no. 4 (July-August 2006): 64-5.

Daily, Thomas V. "Renewed Sense of Identity and Mission." *Origins* 27, no. 4 (June 12, 1997): 55-61.

Danneels, Godfried. "Healthcare and Catholic Identity in the Universal Church." *Health Progress* 68, no. 8 (October 1987): 35-40.

D'Antonio, William V. *American Catholics Today: New Realities of Their Faith and Their Church.* Lanham, Md: Rowman & Littlefield Publishers, 2007.

Dolan, Jay P. "The Church and America." *Health Progress* 83, no. 4 (July-August 2002): 37-41, 62.

Dulles, Avery. *Models of the Church.* Rev. ed. New York, N.Y.: Image Press, 2002.

Egan, Peggy. "Health Care and the Global Community." *Health Progress* 87, no. 4 (July-August 2006): 29-32.

Euart, Sharon. "The Role of the Bishop." *Health Progress* 86, no. 5 (September-October 2005): 38-9.

Evashwick, Connie J. "Integrating Housing and Healthcare." *Health Progress* 81, no. 3 (May-June 2000): 40-3, 51.

Fahey, Charles J. "A New Role for the Church." *Health Progress* 79, no. 5 (September-October 1998): 34-7, 51.

Farrell, Kevin J. "What Does It Mean To Be Catholic Enough?" *Origins* 39, no. 11 (August 13, 2009): 189-91.

Fiorenza, Francis Schüssler. "The Church's Religious Identity and Its Social and Political Mission." *Theological Studies* 43, no. 2 (June 1982): 197-225.

Fox, Zeni. "Making All Things New: Catholic Health Care, the Laity, and the Church." *Health Progress* 92, no. 5 (September-October 2011): 12-5.

_____. "Continuing the Mission: How Do Health Care Leaders Keep Catholic Identity Alive in Today's World?" *Health Progress* 89, no. 2 (March-April 2008): 23-36.

Friend, William B. "Reflections on Fostering Catholic Identity." *Health Progress* 66, no. 6 (June 1985): 57-8.

George, Francis Eugene, and John L. Allen. "Cardinal George: On Catholic Identity, Communion and Politics." *National Catholic Reporter* 44, no. 1 (October 26, 2007): 6.

Giganti, Ed. "Leadership and the Core Commitments." *Health Progress* 85, no. 2 (March-April 2004): 10-1.

_____. "Living Our Promises, Acting on Faith." *Health Progress* 82, no. 1 (January-February 2001): 32.

_____. "Living Our Promises, Acting on Faith." *Health Progress* 80, no. 6 (November-December 1999): 52.

Gilden, Julia. "Hospital Mergers Put Catholic Identity to the Test." *National Catholic Reporter* 28 (March 27, 1992): 4.

Glaser, John W. and Brian B. Glaser. "Systemic Reform Is Vital to Our Ministry." *Health Progress* 83, no. 3 (May-June 2002): 16-9.

Gleason, Philip. "What Made Catholic Identity a Problem?" Marianist Award Lecture. Dayton, Ohio: University of Dayton, 1994.

Gottemoeller, Doris. "Preserving Our Catholic Identity." *Health Progress* 80, no. 3 (May-June 1999): 18-21.

Griese, Orville N., Pope John XXIII Medical-Moral Research and Education Center, and United States Catholic Conference. *Catholic Identity in Health Care: Principles and Practice*. Braintree, Mass: Pope John Center, 1987.

Grogan, William, Melanie Morey, and John Piderit. "Modeling Cultural Contours in a Catholic Hospital. A Facility Can Affirm Its Religious Identity by Adopting Religious Practices." *Health Progress* 88, no. 4 (July-August 2007): 28-35.

Hamel, Ron. "Cardinal Is Clear on Role for Bishops." *Health Progress* 92, no. 4 (July-August 2011): 72-9.

_____. "The Stories We Live By." *Health Progress* 89, no. 3 (May-June 2008): 14-5.

_____. "Caring for Catholic Institutions." *New Theology Review* 14, no. 2 (May 2001): 28-38.

Harvey, Thomas J. "Maintaining Catholic Identity in a Pluralistic Society: Some Reflections." *Hospital Progress* 64, no. 1 (January 1983): 48-53.

Haughian, Richard M. "A Shared Vision of the Future." *Health Progress* 85, no. 3 (May-June 2004): 45-9.

Heft, James. "Catholic Universities as Open Circles: Academic Freedom." *Origins* 35, no. 40 (March 23, 2006): 660-2.

Hehir, J. Bryan. "Identity and Institutions." *Health Progress* 89, no. 3 (May-June 2008): 17-23.

Kauffman, Christopher J. *Ministry and Meaning: A Religious History of Catholic Health Care in the United States.* New York, N.Y.: Crossroad Publishing Company, 1995.

Kelly, Gerard. "The Relationship between Mission and Identity: A Case Study from Theological Education." *Australasian Catholic Record* 84, no. 1 (January 2007): 35-44.

Kicanas, Gerald F.. "Creating an Ecclesial Culture of Dialogue within Catholic Healthcare." *Origins* 41, no. 35 (February 9, 2012): 570-5.

Langan, John. "Reforging Catholic Identity: How Will Non-Catholic Faculty Fit In?" *Commonweal* 127, no. 8 (April 21, 2000): 20-3.

Macchiarola, Frank J. "Catholic Identity." *Commonweal* 126, no. 8 (April 23, 1999): 7-8.

Maddix, Thomas D. "Intuition: The Missing Piece." *Health Progress* 81, no. 5 (September-October 2000): 64, 63.

Malone, James William. "A University's Catholic Identity: Assertive, But Not Sectarian." *Origins* 22, no. 9 (July 23, 1992): 166-8.

_____. "Catholic Universities." *Origins* 23, no. 27 (December 16, 1993): 472-4.

McCormick, Richard A. "The Catholic Hospital Today: Mission Impossible?" *Origins* 24, no. 39 (March 16, 1995): 648-653.

_____. *Health and Medicine in the Catholic Tradition: Tradition in Transition*. New York, N.Y.: Crossroad Publishing Company, 1984.

_____. *The Critical Calling: Reflections on Moral Dilemmas since Vatican II*. Washington, D.C.: Georgetown University Press, 1989.

McConnaha, Scott. "Catholic Teaching and Disparities in Care." *Health Progress* 87, no. 1 (January-February 2006): 46-50.

McGreevy, John T. "Catholic Enough?: Religious Identity at Notre Dame." *Commonweal* 134, no. 16 (September 28, 2007): 7-9.

McGuire, Terrance P., and Mark Tabbut. "Melding Mission and Values." *Health Progress* 81, no. 3 (May-June 2000): 24-6.

Miller, J. Michael. "Catholic Universities and Their Catholic Identity." *Origins* 35, no. 27 (December 15, 2005): 451-8.

Morrisey, Francis G. "What Does Canon Law Say about the Quality of Sponsored Works?" *Health Progress* 88, no. 2 (March-April 2007): 10-1.

_____. "Catholic Identity in a Challenging Environment." *Health Progress* 80, no. 6 (November-December 1999): 38-42.

_____. "Alienation and Administration." *Health Progress* 79, no. 5 (September-October 1998): 24.

Mudd, John O. "From CEO to Mission Leader." *Health Progress* 86, no. 5 (September-October 2005): 25-7.

Nairn, Thomas. "Not Unique, Not Distinct – Yet Catholic?: Integrity Is Key." *Health Progress* 92, no. 4 (July-August 2011): 104-6.

National Conference of Catholic Bishops. *Health and Health Care: A Pastoral Letter of the American Catholic Bishops.* 1981. Reprint, Washington, D.C.: USCCB Publishing, 2003.

Neale, Ann. "Catholic Identity: Realized in Conversation." *Health Progress* 78, no. 2 (March-April 1997): 28-30.

Nelson, Sioban. "Invisible Radicals." *Health Progress* 84, no. 2 (March-April 2003): 27-37, 65.

Niederauer, George H. "Charity and the Identity of the Local Church." *Origins* 35, no. 37 (March 2, 2006): 609-12.

O'Donohoe, James A. "Pluralism, Loss of Identity: Critical Issues in Catholic Health Care." *Hospital Progress* 61, no. 11 (November 1980): 48-51.

O'Rourke, Kevin D. "Canon Law and the Ethical and Religious Directives." *Health Progress* 87, no. 3 (May-June 2006): 42-3.

_____. "Catholic Identity in Health Care." *Health Progress* 69, no. 7 (September 1988): 86.

O'Rourke, Kevin D., Thomas Kopfensteiner, and Ron Hamel. "The ERDs: A Brief History." *Health Progress* 82, no. 6 (November-December 2001): 18-21.

O'Toole, Brian. "The Hallmark of Catholic Identity." *Health Progress* 89, no. 3 (May-June 2008): 46-51.

Ouellet, Marc. "The Ecclesiology of Communion, 50 Years after the Opening of Vatican Council II." Address, International Theology Symposium, Maynooth, Ontario: St. Patrick's College, June 7, 2012, http://www.catholicculture.org/culture/library/view.cfm?recnum=9968.

Pellegrino, Edmund D. "Catholic Identity in Medical Schools." *Health Progress* 74, no. 1 (January-February 1993): 70-3.

_____. "Evangelization and the Catholic Identity of Medical Schools." *Linacre Quarterly* 60, no. 11 (1993): 7-21.

Perry, Beth. "Living Our Mission." *Health Progress* 84, no. 3 (May-June 2003): 16-19, 51.

Pilarczyk, Daniel Edward. "Strong Catholic Identity Key to Effective Health Care Apostolate." *Hospital Progress* 61, no. 11 (November 1980): 46-7.

Place, Michael D. "Agenda for the Strong at Heart. Facing the Challenges Ahead Will Require Recommitment to Our Right To Serve in a Manner Faithful to Our Identity." *Health Progress* 83, no. 4 (July-August 2002): 30-4, 58.

_____. "Catholic Identity: A Unifying Force." *Health Progress* 80, no. 2 (March-April 1999): 10, 14.

Porter, Robert G. "The Essence of Catholic Health Care." *Health Progress* 81, no. 6 (November-December 2000): 14-20.

Rigali, Justin F. "The Catholic Identity of Catholic Charities." *Origins* 31, no. 31 (January 17, 2002): 520-4.

Rinere, Elissa. "Catholic Identity and the Use of the Name 'Catholic'." *Jurist* 62, no. 1 (2002): 131-58.

Roberts, Tom. "Authority and Identity." *National Catholic Reporter* 47, no. 7 (January 21, 2011): 1.

Rodriquez, Oscar. "Catholic Health Care's Witness." *Origins* 35, no. 5 (June 16, 2005): 69-74.

Rymarz, Richard. "John Paul II and the 'New Evangelization': Origins and Meaning." *Australian eJournal of Theology* 15, no. 1 (2010): 1-22. http://aejt.com.au/__data/assets/pdf_file/0009/225396/Rymarcz_evangelization_GH.pdf

Schindler, Thomas F. "What Makes Catholic Managed Care Catholic?" *Health Progress* 76, no. 5 (June 1995): 52-4.

Skylstad, William S. "Serving God's People." *Health Progress* 89, no. 3 (May-June 2008): 24-5.

_____. "Catholic Health Care's Identity and Integrity." *Origins* 36, no. 6 (June 22, 2006): 85-93.

Smith, Patricia. "Canon Law Is Flexible and Adjustable." *Health Progress* 86, no. 6 (November-December 2005): 50-1.

Sullivan, Joseph M. "Ministering Together." *Health Progress* 83, no. 4 (July-August 2002): 42-4, 62.

Sulmasy, Daniel P. "Can Medical Schools Be Catholic?" *Health Progress* 84, no. 4 (July-August 2003): 10-13, 50.

Taylor, Carol. "The Buck Stops Here." *Health Progress* 82, no. 5 (September-October 2001): 37-40.

Timm, Kami. "An Examination of Conscience: The Catholic Identity of Catholic Health Care." *Health Progress* 93, no. 1 (January-February 2012): 6-11.

Travaline, John M. "Catholic Identity in Catholic Health-Care Institutions: Are We Doing Enough?" *Linacre Quarterly* 77, no. 2 (May 2010): 136-8.

United States Conference of Catholic Bishops. *The Ethical and Religious Directives for Catholic Health Care Services.* 5th ed. Washington, D.C.: USCCB Publishing, 2009.

van Beeck, Frans Jozef. *Catholic Identity after Vatican II: Three Types of Faith in the One Church.* Campion book. Chicago, Il: Loyola University Press, 1985.

Vowell, Thomas H. "Preserving Catholic Identity in Mergers." *Health Progress* 73, no. 3 (March 1992): 28-33.

Weakland, Rembert G. *All God's People: Catholic Identity after the Second Vatican Council.* New York, N.Y.: Paulist Press, 1985.

Weber, Leonard J. "Medical Waste and Healthcare Ethics." *Health Progress* 81, no. 1 (January-February 2000): 26-8, 32.

Weisenbeck, Marlene. "Understanding Charism." *Health Progress* 89, no. 6 (November-December 2008): 16-7.

White, Kenneth R. "Hospitals Sponsored by the Roman Catholic Church: Separate, Equal, and Distinct?" *The Milbank Quarterly* 78, no. 2 (June 2000): 213-239.

Wilson, Rose and Thomas F. Schindler. "Traditions in Transition: What Does It Mean to Be a Catholic Health Care Facility Today?" *Health Progress* 71, no. 8 (October 1990): 26-31.

Wood, Glenn G. "Should We Be Concerned about the Content of Mission Statements for Christian Hospitals?" *Christian Bioethics* 7, no. 1 (April 1, 2001): 105-15.

Wright, Corinne, and Rosalie M. Mirenda. "Using Nursing Model To Affirm Catholic Identity." *Health Progress* 68, no. 2 (March 1987): 63-7.

Wuerl, Donald W. "Catholic Health Ministry in Transition." *Health Progress* 80, no. 3 (May-June 1999): 14.

_____. "Solidarity between Bishops and Catholic Institutions." *Origins* 39, no. 4 (June 4, 2009): 49-50.

_____. "The Marks of a Catholic College or University." *Origins* 37, no. 37 (February 28, 2008): 592-6.

THE PRINCIPLE OF MORAL COOPERATION

"Bishop Warns City on 'Cooperation with Evil'." *Christian Century* 121, no. 12 (June 15, 2004): 14.

"Interreligious Assembly at Vatican Calls for Cooperation." *America* 181, no. 15 (November 13, 1999): 5.

"Partnering with Other-Than-Catholic Organizations." *Health Progress* 79, no. 4 (July-August 1998): 21.

"'Pro-choice' Officials Risk Cooperation in Grave Evil." *Our Sunday Visitor* 93, no. 10 (July 4, 2004): 8.

"The Limits of Catholic Cooperation." *Christian Century* 63, no. 20 (May 15, 1946): 611-18.

Arias, Joseph M., and Basil Cole. "The Vademecum and Cooperation in Condomistic Intercourse." *National Catholic Bioethics Quarterly* 11, no. 2 (Summer 2011): 301-28.

Barker, Mark J. "Material Cooperation with Abortion: A Test Case." *Homiletic and Pastoral Review* 109, no. 8 (May 2009): 67-70.

Benedict XVI. "The Co-Responsibility of the Laity." *Origins* 42, no. 16 (September 20, 2012): 254-5.

_____. "A New Spirit of Cooperation and Trust." *Osservatore Romano* 2239, no. 10/11 (March 28, 2012).

_____. "Dialogue and Fraternal Cooperation on the Way toward Unity." *Osservatore Romano* 2148, no. 6 (June 9, 2010).

_____. "Religion and Culture for Cooperation between Peoples." *Osservatore Romano* 2145, no. 6 (May 19, 2010).

Bernardin, Joseph L. "Catholic Institutions and Their Identity." *Origins* 21, no. 2 (May 23, 1991): 33-6.

Blanshard, Paul. "The Catholic Price for Cooperation." *Christian Century* 66, no. 18 (May 4, 1949): 557-9.

Callahan, Sidney. "Cooperating with Evil." *Health Progress* 70, no. 4 (May 1989): 12-4.

Cataldo, Peter J., and John M. Haas. "Institutional Cooperation: The ERDs." *Health Progress* 83, no. 6 (November-December 2002): 49-60.

Cataldo, Peter J. "Compliance with Contraceptive Insurance Mandates: Licit or Illicit Cooperation in Evil?" *National Catholic Bioethics Quarterly* 4, no. 1 (Spring 2004): 103-30.

_____. "A Cooperation Analysis of Embryonic Stem Cell Research." *National Catholic Bioethics Quarterly* 2, no. 1 (Spring 2002): 35-41.

Catholic Health Association. *Report on a Theological Dialogue on the Principle of Cooperation*. St. Louis, Mo: Catholic Health Association, 2007.

Catholic Medical Association and National Catholic Bioethics Center. *A Catholic Guide to Ethical Clinical Research*. Philadelphia, Pa: Catholic Medical Association, 2008.

Deets, M. King. "The Board's Role in Meaningful Collaboration." *Health Progress* 72, no. 6 (June 1991): 46-8.

De George, Richard T. "The Moral Responsibility of the Hospital." *Journal of Medicine and Philosophy* 7, no. 1 (February 1982): 87-100.

Dewan, Lawrence. "Wisdom, Law, and Virtue: Essays in Thomistic Ethics." *Moral Philosophy & Moral Theology*. 1st ed. New York, N.Y.: Fordham University Press, 2008.

Ernst, Harold E. "Catholic Politicians, Voters, and Cooperation in Evil: A Response to Rev. Thomas Kopfensteiner." *Chicago Studies* 44, no. 2 (Summer 2005): 203-18.

Fisher, Anthony. *Catholic Bioethics for a New Millennium*. Cambridge, UK; New York, N.Y.: Cambridge University Press, 2012.

_____. "Co-operation in Evil." *Catholic Medical Quarterly* 44, no. 3 (February 1994): 15-22.

Fogarty, Gerald P. "Vatican-American Relations: Cooperation or Conspiracy?" *America* 166, no. 12 (April 11, 1992): 289-93.

Furton, Edward James, Peter J. Cataldo, Albert S. Moraczewski, and National Catholic Bioethics Center. *Catholic Health Care Ethics: A Manual for Practitioners*. 2nd ed. Philadelphia, Pa: National Catholic Bioethics Center, 2009.

Gallagher, John A. "A Theological Reflection on the Principle of Cooperation and the Catholic Health Ministry." *Health Care Ethics USA* 21, no. 1 (Winter 2013): 2-9.

Grisez, Germaine. *The Way of the Lord Jesus*, 3. Quincy, Il: Franciscan Press, 1997.

Haas, John. "There Are No 'Prohibited Services': Getting the Language Right." *Ethics and Medics* 35, no. 3 (March 2010): 1-2.

Hamel, Ron. "Cooperation: A Principle Reflects Reality." *Health Progress* 93, no. 5 (September-October 2012): 80-82.

_____ and Michael R. Panicola. "Cooperating with Philanthropic Organizations: How to Assess the Moral Permissibility of a Catholic Health Care Organization's Involvement." *Health Progress* 89, no. 2 (March-April 2008): 49-55.

Happel, Stephen Paul. "Rites of Initiation and the Politics of Cooperation." *Liturgy* 7, no. 4 (1988): 27-31.

John Paul II. "Jubilee Calls for Effort and Cooperation." *Osservatore Romano* 1626 (January 19, 2000): 3.

_____. "Church-State Co-Operation Benefits All." *Osservatore Romano* 1536 (April 8, 1998): 6.

_____. "Cooperation." *Osservatore Romano 36* (September 8, 1993): 11.

Kaveny, M. Cathleen. "Appropriation of Evil: Cooperation's Mirror Image." *Theological Studies* 61, no. 2 (June 2000): 280-313.

──── and James F. Keenan. "Ethical Issues in Health-Care Restructuring." *Theological Studies* 56, no. 1 (March 1995): 136-150.

Keenan, James F. "Developments in Bioethics from the Perspective of HIV/AIDS." *Cambridge Quarterly of Healthcare Ethics* 14, no. 4 (October 2005): 416-23.

_____. "Collaboration and Cooperation in Catholic Health Care." *Australasian Catholic Record* 77 (April 2000): 163-74.

_____. "Institutional Cooperation and the Ethical and Religious Directives." *The Linacre Quarterly* 64, no. 3 (August 1997): 53-76.

_____. "Prophylactics, Toleration and Cooperation: Contemporary Problems and Traditional Principles." *International Philosophical Quarterly* 29, no. 2 (June 1989): 205-20.

_____. Jon D. Fuller, Lisa Sowle Cahill, and Kevin Kelly, eds. *Catholic Ethicists on HIV/AIDS Prevention.* New York, N.Y.: Continuum, 2000.

_____. and Thomas R. Kopfensteiner. "The Principle of Cooperation." *Health Progress* 76, no. 3 (April 1995): 23-7.

———— and Kevin D. O'Rourke. 1998. "Cooperation and 'Hard Cases.'" *Ethics and Medics* 23, no. 9 (September 1998): 3-4.

Kissell, Judith Lee. "Cooperation with Evil: Its Contemporary Relevance." *Linacre Quarterly* 62, no. 1 (February 1995): 33-45.

Kopfensteiner, Thomas. "The Man with a Ladder: Politicians, Voters and the Principle of Cooperation." *America* 191, no. 13 (November 1, 2004): 9-11.

————. "The Meaning and Role of Duress in the Cooperation in Wrongdoing." *Linacre Quarterly* 70, no. 2 (May 2003): 150-8.

————. "Responsibility and Cooperation: Evaluating Partnerships among Health Care Providers." *Health Progress* 83, no. 6 (November-December 2002): 40.

Latkovic, Mark S. "Pro-Life Nurses and Cooperation in Abortion: Ordinary Care or Extraordinary Intervention?" *National Catholic Bioethics Quarterly* 4, no. 1 (Spring 2004): 89-102.

Lewis, Brian. "Cooperation Revisited." *Australasian Catholic Record* 77, no. 2 (April 2000): 158-62.

McDermott, John A. "Catholic-Protestant Cooperation". *Christian Century* 78, no. 32 (August 9, 1961): 959-60.

Morrisey, Francis G. "Restructuring Systems: A Call for Dialogue." *Health Progress* 94, no. 1 (January-February 2013): 66-7.

Mulholland, Edward. "Lobbying for Life and Death at the UN." *National Catholic Register* 75 (April 4, 1999): 9.

Murray, John Courtney. "Cooperation: Some Current Views." *Theological Studies* 4, no. 1 (March 1943): 100-11.

_____. "Intercredal Cooperation: Its Theory and Its Organization." *Theological Studies* 4, no. 2 (June 1943): 257-86.

Nairn, Thomas. "Just Because It Shocks Doesn't Make It Scandal." *Health Progress* 93, no. 6 (November-December 2012): 72-5.

Napier, Stephen E. "Catholic Hospitals, Institutional Review Boards, and Cooperation." *National Catholic Bioethics Quarterly* 11, no. 2 (Summer 2011): 257-66.

National Catholic Bioethics Center. "Cooperating with Non-Catholic Partners. Statement on Cooperation by the Ethicists of the National Catholic Bioethics Center. An Examination of the Fundamental Principles." *Ethics and Medics* 23, no. 11 (November 1998): 1-4.

Nienstedt, John C. "Reexamining the ERDs on Cooperation." *Ethics and Medics* 26, no. 5 (May 2001): 1-2.

_____. "Catholic Health Care Cooperation: Why Rewrite the Ethical and Religious Directives?" *Linacre Quarterly* 68, no. 2 (May 2011): 97-100.

O'Rourke, Kevin D. "Catholic Health Care and Sterilization. The 'Principle of Cooperation' Provides the Necessary Ethical Guidelines." *Health Progress* 83, no. 6 (November-December 2002): 43-8, 60.

O'Rourke, Kevin D., and Philip Boyle. *Medical Ethics: Sources of Catholic Teachings*. 4th ed. Washington, D.C.: Georgetown University Press, 2011.

O'Rourke, Kevin D., Thomas Kopfensteiner, and Ron Hamel. "A Brief History: A Summary of the Development of the Ethical and Religious Directives for Catholic Health Care Services." *Health Progress* 82, no. 6 (November-December 2001): 18-21.

Panicola, Michael R., and Ron Hamel. "Conscience, Cooperation, and Full Disclosure." *Health Progress* 87, no. 1 (January-February 2006): 52-9.

Parsons, Wilfrid. "Intercredal Cooperation in the Papal Documents." *Theological Studies* 4, no. 2 (June 1943): 159-82.

Pevtzow, Lisa. "Even at a Distance, Catholic Hospitals' 'Cooperation with Evil' Disturbs Some Ethicists." *National Catholic Register* 74 (January 11, 1998): 1.

Pint, Rose Mary. "Risks and Responsibilities." *Health Progress* 72, no. 5 (June 1991): 36-8.

Popovici, Alice. "Religion at Heart of Questions over Hospital Merger." *National Catholic Reporter* 47, no. 23 (September 2, 2011): 1.

Ratzinger, Joseph. "Facilitating Moral Evil." *Crisis* 6, no. 8 (September 1988): 41.

Riga, Peter John. "Public Funding of Abortions and Catholic Cooperation." *Priest* 41 (July 1985): 14-8.

Rudin, James. "Health-Care Cooperation." *Catholic International* 3 (July 1992): 614-5.

Scarnecchia, D. Brian. "Bioethics, Law, and Human Life Issues: A Catholic Perspective on Marriage, Family, Contraception, Abortion, Reproductive Technology, and Death and Dying." *Catholic Social Thought* 2. Lanham, Md: Scarecrow Press, 2010.

Sigmond, Robert M. "Cooperation, Competition, Regulation: Health Care System's Balancing Act." *Hospital Progress* 62, no. 3 (March 1981): 32-5.

Smith, Janet E. and Christopher Robert Kaczor. *Life Issues, Medical Choices: Questions and Answers for Catholics*. Cincinnati, Ohio: St. Anthony Messenger Press, 2007.

Smith, Russell. "Formal and Material Cooperation." *Ethics and Medics* 20, no. 6 (June 1995): 1-2.

Smith, Russell. "The Principles of Cooperation in Catholic Thought." In *The Fetal Tissue Issue: Medical and Ethical Aspects*, edited by Peter J. Cataldo and Albert S. Moraczewski. Braintree, Mass: The Pope John XXIII Medical-Moral Research and Education Center, 1994, 81-92.

_____. "Duress and Cooperation." *Ethics and Medics* 21, no. 11 (November 1996): 1-2.

Sulmasy, Daniel P. "Institutional Conscience and Moral Pluralism in Health Care." *New Theology Review* 10, no. 4 (1997): 5-12.

Szoka, Edmund Casimir. "Formal and Material Cooperation in Moral Theology." *Origins* 12, no. 42 (March 31, 1983): 679.

United States Catholic Conference, "Faithful Citizenship." (video). Washington, D.C.: United States Catholic Conference and Golden Dome Productions. 2000.

Watt, Helen. *Cooperation, Complicity, and Conscience: Problems in Health Care, Science, Law, and Public Policy*. Oxford, England: Linacre Center, 2006.

Weber, Leonard J. "The Business of Ethics." *Health Progress* 71, no. 1 (January 1990): 75.

White, Kenneth R. "Hospitals Sponsored by the Roman Catholic Church: Separate, Equal, and Distinct?" *The Milbank Quarterly* 78, no. 2 (June 2000): 213-239.

Whitehead, Kenneth D., ed. *Conscience, Cooperation & Complicity: Proceedings from the 31st Annual Convention of the Fellowship of Catholic Scholars.* Scranton, Pa: University of Scranton Press, 2008.

CATHOLIC ECONOMIC THOUGHT AND FOR-PROFIT HEALTH CARE

"Cardinal Opposes Catholic Hospital's Sale to For-Profit Chain." *National Catholic Register* 73 (November 9, 1997): 2.

"Catholic Health Care Rated High." *National Catholic Reporter* (August 20, 2010): 3.

"Hospitals Enter Debate over Catholic Identity." *National Catholic Reporter* 34 (November 7, 1997): 20.

"Outreach Program Serves Rural Hospitals, Businesses." *Hospital Progress* 63, no. 10 (October 1982): 28-9.

"Pope Opposes Usury of Big Business." *Christian Century* 36, no. 33 (August 14, 1919): 6.

"Profit Motive Ignites Debate between Proprietaries, Non-Profits." *Hospital Progress* 62, no. 6 (June 1981): 20-1.

"Queen of For-Profit Hospitals." *Our Sunday Visitor* 87 (May 31, 1998): 4.

*Rethinking the Purpose of Business: Interdisciplinary Essays from the
Catholic Social Tradition.* S.A. Cortright and Michael J. Naughton,
eds. Reviewed by Thomas Storck. *New Oxford Review* 70, no. 9
(October 2003): 45-6.

"Social Accountability: The Next Generation." *Health Progress* 80,
no. 6 (November-December 1999): 12-6.

Abela, Andrew. "Profit Pointers." *National Catholic Register* 87, no. 1
(January 2, 2011): 1-b2.

Ackerman, Todd. "Hospitals Face For-Profit Challenge." *National
Catholic Register* 61 (October 13, 1985): 1.

Albers, John E. "Effects of Changes in Healthcare Delivery on
Catholic Hospitals." *Social Justice Review* 93, no. 3/4 (March 2002):
44-6.

Alford, Helen. "The Responsibilities of Theology to Business (or the
Responsibilities of the Butcher, the Baker, and the Imagemaker)."
New Blackfriars 81, no. 1 (2000): 27-35.

Arbuckle, Gerald A. "Nine Axioms for Success in Mergers: Health
Care Leaders Must Take Great Care with the Cultural Factors
Involved." *Health Progress* 84, no. 1 (January-February 2003):
38-42.

_____. "Mission and Business: Resolving the Tension: An Awareness
of the Process of 'Splitting' Can Help Organizations Achieve a
Creative Balance." *Health Progress* 80, no. 5 (September-October
1999): 22.

Arnerich, John Paul. "For Non-Profit Hospitals, a Hard Time from
Feds?" *National Catholic Register* 67 (April 14, 1991): 1.

Barger-Lux, M. "Profit, Technology, and the Loss of Ideals." *Health Progress* 66, no. 7 (September 1985): 88-91.

Barrera, Albino. "Globalization's Shifting Economic and Moral Terrain: Contesting Marketplace Mores." *Theological Studies*, 69, no. 2 (June 2008): 290-308.

Barrows, Stephen Paul. "Labor Economics and the Development of Papal Social Encyclicals." *Journal of Markets & Morality* 14, no. 1 (March 1, 2011): 7-22.

Benedict XVI. "Blessed Are the Peacemakers." Message for the World Day of Peace, January 1, 2013.

_____. "Businesses Have a Social Responsibility." *Osservatore Romano* 2132 (February 17, 2010): 12.

_____. "Beyond the Logic of Profit Lies Charity." *Osservatore Romano* 2132 (February 17, 2010): 7.

Bernardin, Joseph. "The Case for Not-For-Profit Health Care." *Origins* 24, no. 32 (January 26, 1995): 538-42.

Birchall, Johnston, and Richard E. Simmons. "The Involvement of Members in the Governance of Large-Scale Co-Operative and Mutual Businesses." *Review of Social Economy* 62, no. 4 (December 2004): 487-515.

Bole, William. "Struggles of Modern Catholic Executives." *Catholic Digest* 70, no. 6 (April 2006): 72-7.

_____. "Wages of Justice." *Our Sunday Visitor* 92, no. 18 (August 31, 2003): 9-10.

_____. "Shareholders Speak Out, and God Gets a Pink Slip." *Our Sunday Visitor* 90, no. 34 (December 23, 2001): 3.

_____. "Profits from Heaven." *Our Sunday Visitor* 84 (April 21, 1996): 16-7.

_____. "Putting People before Profits." *Our Sunday Visitor* 85 (June 16, 1996): 6-7.

Boswell, Jonathan S. "Social Cooperation in Economic Systems; A Business History Approach." *Review of Social Economy* 38, no. 10 (1980): 155-77.

Bouchard, Charles. "The Good, the Bad and the Profitable: Morality, Spirituality, and Business." *Listening* 39, no. 2 (Spring 2004): 407-19.

_____. "The Barons of Bankruptcy: Capitalism without a Conscience." *Liguorian* 90, no. 9 (November 2002): 24-7.

Brown, Grattan Taylor. "The Social Responsibility of Catholic Health Care Institutions." *National Catholic Bioethics Quarterly* 8, no. 4 (December 2008): 697-708.

Bruni, Luigino and Amelia J. Uelmen. "What Is the Economy of Communion?" *Living City* 46 (June 2007): 12.

Carroll, Kelly A. "Can For-profit Catholic Health Care Get the Mission Right?" *Health Progress* 93, no. 3 (May-June 2012): 49-59.

Casey, Juliana and William J. Flynn. "Not-for-profits Face Challenges." *Health Progress* 68, no. 7 (July 1987): 76-7.

Catholic Health Association. "Commitment to the Poor and Business Development." *Health Progress* 84, no. 6 (November-December 2003): 42.

Catholic Health Association. "Mission-Driven Market Strategies: Lessons from the Field." *Health Progress* 79, no. 4 (July-August 1998): 50-3.

Celichowski, John. "Health Care as a Human Right, a Ministry and a Business." *Origins* 34, no. 3 (June 3, 2004): 45-8.

Clark, Charles and Michael Andres. "Economic Life in Catholic Social Thought and Economic Theory." In *Catholic Social Thought: American Reflections on the Compendium*, edited by D. Paul Sullins and Anthony J. Blasi. Washington, D.C.: Lexington Books, 2009, 77-99.

_____. "Catholic Social Thought and the Economic Problem" *OIKONOMIA* 1 (February 2001): 6-18.

Clifton, James. "Can For-Profit Hospitals Be Catholic? Yes, Hospital's Care of Indigent Has Grown." *National Catholic Reporter* 34 (December 5, 1997): 20-1.

Clinton, Hillary Rodham. "Not-For-Profits' Role in a Reformed System." *Health Progress* 75, no. 5 (June 1994): 22-6.

Cochran, Clarke E. and Kenneth R. White. "Does Catholic Sponsorship Matter?" *Health Progress* 83, no. 1 (January-February 2002): 14.

Coday, Dennis. "Faith Based Insurance Offered." *National Catholic Reporter* (October 15, 2004): 3.

Coleman, Andrea Y. "Mission: Good Business Practice Enhances Mission." *Health Progress* 92, no. 2 (March–April 2011): 56-9.

Connor, James L. "Beware of False Profits: A Christian Guide to Business." *Liguorian* 98, no. 7 (September 2010): 20-4.

_____. "How to Heal Managed Care: Health Care Is Not a Business." *Commonweal* 127, no. 4 (February 25, 2000): 17-8.

Cope, Francine, Norma Hagenow, and Mehmet Kocakulah."The True Costs of Nursing Care." *Health Progress* 71, no. 10 (December 1990): 48-51.

Coston, Carol. "Worker-Owned Cooperatives: A New Approach for American Business." *America* 152, no. 23 (June 15, 1985): 489-91.

Coverdale, John F. "Why the Bottom Line Is Not the Bottom Line: John Paul II's Concept of Business." *Journal of Catholic Legal Studies* 45, no. 2 (2007): 473-521.

Curley, John E., Jr. "For-Profit Chains Seeking To Buy Catholic Hospitals." *Origins* 25, no. 5 (June 15, 1995): 78-9.

Czarnetzki, John M. "Catholic Theory of Corporate Law." *Catholic Social Science Review* 12 (2007): 69-82.

Davis, John B. "The Science of Happiness and the Marginalization of Ethics." *Review of Social Economy* 45, no. 12 (1987): 298-312.

de Blois, Jean. "Can For-Profit Hospitals Be Catholic? No, Healthcare Is a Basic Human Right." *National Catholic Reporter* 34 (December 5, 1997): 20-1.

DeMeo, Doug. "Prudential Investment: Can Catholic Institutions Do Well While Doing Good?" *America* 201, no. 11 (October 26, 2009): 10-4.

DiPietro, Melanie and Alison Sulentic. "SSM Health Care: The Integration of Catholic Social Thought Values in a Modern Health Care System." *Journal of Catholic Legal Studies* 46, no. 2 (2007): 175-209.

Enderle, Georges. "Has Business Been Good?" *U.S. Catholic* 69, no. 5 (May 2004): 18-22.

Fairchild, Daniel R. "Economic Efficiency, Growth, and the Catholic Vision of Economic Justice." *Logos* 6, no. 1 (2003): 100-19.

Fassel, Diane. "Effective Organizations Are Driven by Values: Survey Data Show that Values-Driven Catholic Health Care Facilities Are Effective Facilities." *Health Progress* 83, no. 5 (September-October 2002): 35.

Feuerherd, Joe. "Catholic Hospitals to Report on 'Community Benefit'." *National Catholic Reporter* 42, no. 41 (September 22, 2006): 5.

_____. "How Corporate? How Catholic?" *National Catholic Reporter* (December 23, 2005): 5-6.

Filteau, Jerry. "Measuring Quality of Care: Study Ranks Catholic Health Systems Best, For-Profits Worst." *National Catholic Reporter* 46, no. 26 (October 15, 2010): 3-3a.

Finn, Daniel, ed. *The True Wealth of Nations: Catholic Social Thought and Economic Life.* New York, N.Y.: Oxford University Press, 2010.

Finn, Seamus. "The Path to Holiness and Wholeness: Mission in the Marketplace." *Origins* 41, no. 1 (May 12, 2011): 12-5.

Fitzpatrick, James K. "The Dilemma of Catholic Corporate Executives." *New Oxford Review* 63, no. 12 (1996): 20-2.

Ford, Mary Kevin. "A Ministry, Not a Business." *Health Progress* 77, no. 5 (September-October 1996): 64.

Foster, David. "Differences in Health System Quality Performance by Ownership." *Thomson-Reuters* (August 9, 2010).

Frayne, Laurence J. "New Dawn for Not-For-Profit Providers." *Health Progress* 67, no. 8 (October 1986): 58-60.

Fried, J. "The New Health Care for Profit." *Health Progress* 65, no. 9 (September 1984): 81.

Gaspari, Antonio. "Debate: Between Profit and Poverty." *Inside the Vatican* 5, no. 6 (1997): 54-7.

Gottemoeller, Doris. "For Profit and Catholic? How Would the Ministry Fare?" *Health Progress* 93, no. 4 (July-August 2012): 31-5.

Graves, Jim. "Radical Business Makeover: Rethinking the Balance of Profits & People Along Lines of Pope Benedict XVI's Social Encyclical." *Our Sunday Visitor* 99, no. 4 (May 23, 2010): 6.

Hamel, Ron P. "Fostering an Ethical Culture: Rules Are Not Enough." *Health Progress* 90, no. 1 (January-February 2009): 10-2.

_____. "Organizational Ethics: Why Bother?" *Health Progress* 87, no. 6 (November-December 2006): 4-5.

Hammond, Sheila. "Nurturing a Catholic Vision in a For-Profit Hospital: Saint Louis University Hospital Fulfills a Promise to Carry Forward the Catholic Mission." *Health Progress* 90, no. 3 (May-June 2009): 57-9.

Heiser, W. C. "Great Giveaway: Reclaiming the Mission of the Church from Big Business, Parachurch Organizations, Psychotherapy, Consumer Capitalism." *Theology Digest* 53, no. 1 (Spring 2006): 69.

Herrera, David. "Mondragón: A For-Profit Organization that Embodies Catholic Social Thought." *Review of Business* 25, no. 1 (Winter 2004): 56-69. Also available at: http://www.stthomas.edu/cathstudies/cst/conferences/bilbao/papers/Herrera.pdf.

Hiebert-White, Jane. "Hospital Conversions: Does Not-For-Profit Status Matter?" *Health Progress* 78, no. 2 (March-April 1997): 10-12.

_____. "Market Transformation: Will Not-For-Profit Providers Survive?" *Health Progress* 77, no. 3 (May-June 1996): 10-12.

Humphrey, Michael. "Value People over Profits, Bishop Urges." *National Catholic Reporter* 44, no. 18 (May 2, 2008): 19.

Jacobsen, Brent, and Jeanne Fitzgerald. "Study Fails To Prove For-Profits' Superiority." *Health Progress* 68, no. 3 (April 1987): 32-7.

John Paul II. "Putting People before Profit Builds a Better World." *Osservatore Romano* 1862 (September 29, 2004): 5.

_____. "Business Executives' Duty in an Age of Globalization." *The Pope Speaks* 49, no. 5 (September 2004): 276-7.

_____. "Charity in a World Obsessed by Profit." *National Catholic Register* 78, no. 8 (February 24, 2002): 5.

_____. "Christian Executives Must Stress 'Being' over 'Having'." *Osservatore Romano* 1835 (March 17, 2005): 3.

_____. "The Profit Motive Behind Too Much Medical Research." *Origins* 31, no. 45 (April 25, 2002): 754-5.

_____. "The Holy Father Addressed the Business Leaders of Naples Stressing that the Common Good Is Served when Moral Criteria, Not Only Economic Ones, Underlie All Concrete Business Decisions." *The Pope Speaks* 36 (July 1991): 193-6.

_____. "Address of the Holy Father to Members of the International Christian Union of Business Directors, Stating that the Treatment of the Workers and Questionable Activities in the World of Work Must Be Renounced." *The Pope Speaks* 36 (September 1991): 261-3.

_____. "The Holy Father Addressed a Group of Italian Catholic Business Men and Women on Their Role in Promoting Social Justice and Putting the Principles of the Church's Social Doctrine, Rerum Novarum, into Practice." *Osservatore Romano* 1187 (April 22, 1991): 2.

_____. "Address of the Holy Father to the Mexican Business Leaders in Durango's Ricardo Castro Theater Stressing Market Ethics and Consideration for the Poor." *Osservatore Romano* 1141 (May 21, 1990): 6.

_____. "Message to American Business Executives Saying that the Principle of Human Dignity Should Govern Economic Activity." *Osservatore Romano* 933 (April 21, 1986): 2.

_____. "Address to Workers in Sydney, Australia, Saying that the Worker Is Always More Important than both Profits and Machines." *Origins* 16, no. 26 (December 11, 1986): 482-4.

_____. "Discourse to Workers, Contractors and Business Executives in Venice, Italy, about the Need for New Forms of Solidarity among Workers." *Osservatore Romano*. 898 (August 12, 1985): 9-10.

_____. "Address to Representatives of the Industrial Classes in Bari, Italy, Saying that Man, the Image of God, Comes before All Profit." *Osservatore Romano* 826 (March 20, 1984): 6-7.

_____. "Discourse to Business Men and Economic Managers Saying that Man and His Values Are the Principle and Aim of Economics." *Documentation Catholique* 80 (July 3, 1983): 659-62.

Johnson, Tracy K. "Revenue Enhancement Strategies: Last in a Series Examining Revenue Growth Strategies in a Difficult Health Care Market." *Health Progress* 83, no. 3 (May-June 2002): 23-6.

Jones, Arthur. "The Endless Rationalization of Profit." *National Catholic Reporter* 36 (December 10, 1999): 19.

Kaiser, Leland R. "Survival Strategies for Not-For-Profit Hospitals." *Hospital Progress* 64, no. 12 (December 1983): 40-6.

Karam, Judith Ann. "Living the Mission in a Business Model of Health: Sisters of Charity Health System." *Health Progress* 89, no. 3 (May-June 2008): 38-9.

Liechty, Daniel. "Redeeming Marketplace Medicine: A Theology of Healthcare." *Journal of Religion and Health* 39, no. 3 (September 2000): 285-6.

Longley, Clifford. "Gift Means Giving Up the Pursuit of Every Last Morsel of Profit." *Tablet* 263, no. 8805 (August 15, 2009): 5.

Lustig, B. Andrew. "Managed Care, Catholic Vision, and the Claims of Justice." *Christian Bioethics* 6, no. 3 (December 2000): 219-300.

Luxmoore, Jonathan. "Vatican's UN Observer Condemns Multinational Companies." *Tablet* 265, no. 8900 (June 18, 2011): 28.

Lysaught, M. Therese. "Reverse Innovation from the Least of Our Neighbors." *Health Progress* 94, no. 1 (January-February 2013): 45-52.

MacEóin, Gary. "Another Catholic Hospital Goes For-Profit." *National Catholic Reporter* 34 (September 18, 1998): 5.

Macey, Jonathan R. "A Close Read of an Excellent Commentary on Dodge v Ford." *Virginia Law and Business Review*, 3 (Spring 2008): 177-190.

Maddix, Tom. "The Challenge of Resource Allocation: Wise Decisions Require Organizations To Ask Difficult Questions." *Health Progress* 86, no. 4 (July-August 2005): 60-2.

Mahar, Maggie. "How U.S. Health Care Mirrors the Contradictions Ingrained in the Minds and Souls of America's Citizens." *Health Beat Blog*, September 17, 2008. http://www.healthbeatblog.com/2008/09/how-us-health-c/.

Maloney, Oliver. "Justice Day-By-Day: Fair Profit." *Furrow* 40, no. 8 (August 1989): 467-70.

Martin, Diarmud. "Catholic Social Teaching and Human Work: The 25th Anniversary of *Laborem Exercens.*" *Journal of Catholic Social Thought* 6, no. 1 (January 2009): 5-17.

Martin, Michelle. "Is a Business Model Right for the Church?" *Our Sunday Visitor* 94, no. 24 (October 9, 2005): 3.

McClintock, Brent. "The Multinational Corporation and Social Justice." *Review of Social Economy* 57, no. 4 (July 1999): 507-22.

McConnaha, Scott. "Who Cares about Ethics?: Five Ethicists and Five Executives Discuss the Importance of Ethical Guidance in Catholic Health Care Today." *Health Progress* 85, no. 3 (May-June 2004): 15-22.

McCormick, Patrick T. "Not for Profit: Why Democracy Needs the Humanities." *US Catholic* 75, no. 10 (October 2010): 42.

McDonough, Mary J. *Can a Health Care Market Be Moral? A Catholic Vision*. Washington, D.C.: Georgetown University Press, 2007.

McHugh, Frank. "A Century of Catholic Social Teaching." *Priest & People* 5, no. 5 (September-October 1991): 173-7.

McKee, Arnold F. "What Is Just Profit?" *Review of Social Economy* 46 (Summer 1989): 173-84.

Meyer, Donna, and Catherine Rowan. "Using Investments To Work for Community Health." *Health Progress* 88, no. 6 (November-December 2007): 54-8.

Miller, Amata. "Merging with For-Profits: Flawed Strategy." *Health Progress* 77, no. 4 (July-August 1996): 14-7.

Mueller, Celeste M. "Theology Goes to Work: Applying Theological Reflection to the Business of the Day." *Health Progress* 90, no. 4 (July-August 2009): 37-43.

Naughton, Michael J. "The 'Stumbling and Tripping' of Executive Pay." *New Oxford Review* 68, no. 11 (December 2001): 27-32.

Nürnberger, Klaus. "Is the Human Being a Profit and Pleasure Maximiser? The Concept of the *Homo Oeconomicus* in Economic Theory as a Deceptive Norm and Its Theological Demythologisation." *Religion & Theology* 3, no. 3 (August 1996): 218-45.

Pellegrino, Edmund D. "Ethical Issues in Managed Care: A Catholic Christian Perspective." *Christian Bioethics* 3, no. 1 (March 1997): 55-73.

Percy, Anthony. "Private Initiative, Entrepreneurship, and Business in the Teaching of Pius XII." *Journal of Markets & Morality* 7, no. 1 (Spring 2004): 7-25.

Peter, Val J. "Why Preserve the Not-For-Profit Tradition?" *Health Progress* 79, no. 2 (March-April 1998): 80.

Place, Michael D. "Agenda for the Strong at Heart. Facing the Challenges Ahead Will Require Recommitment to Our Right to Serve in a Manner Faithful to Our Identity." *Health Progress* 83, no. 4 (July-August 2002): 30-4, 58.

_____. "Planned Sale of St. Louis University Hospital to For-Profit Chain." *Origins* 27, no. 30 (January 15, 1998): 497.

Popovici, Alice. "A Catholic Foray into For-Profit Health Care." *National Catholic Reporter* (December 17, 2012): 15.

Relman, Arnold S. "Selling to the For-Profits: Undermining the Mission." *Health Progress* 66, no. 7 (September 1985): 81-5.

Rigali, Justin F. "St. Louis University Hospital Sold to For-Profit Corporation." *Origins* 27, no. 38 (March 12, 1998): 629.

_____. "Proposed Sale of Two Catholic Hospitals to For-Profit Chain." *Origins* 27, no. 21 (November 6, 1997): 362-4.

Sinclair, John L. "Mission-Based HR Drives Business Success." *Health Progress* 81, no. 5 (September-October 2000): 28-31.

Sneirson, Judd F. "The Sustainable Corporation and Shareholder Profits." *Wake Forest Law Review* 46 (2011): 541-559.

Stanek, Robert V. "Bridging the Mission-Business Gap in Health Care." *Health Progress* 89, no. 3 (May-June 2008): 35-7.

Stewart, James B. "Building a Cooperative Economy: Lessons from the Black Experience." *Review of Social Economy* 42, no. 3 (December 1984): 360-8.

Stout, Lynn. "Why We Should Stop Teaching Dodge v. Ford." *Virginia Law and Business Review* 3 (Spring 2008): 164-176.

Sullivan, Brian G. "*Laborem Exercens*: A Theological and Philosophical Foundation for Business Ethics." *Listening* 20 (Spring 1985): 128-46.

Talone, Patricia A. "Budgeting as Theological Reflection." *Health Progress* 85, no. 1 (January-February 2004): 14-7.

_____. "A Values-Guided 'Downsizing'." *Health Progress* 83, no. 2 (March-April 2002): 39-42.

Tomasi, Silvano M. "Finances Should Reduce Poverty Not Just Increase Profit." *Osservatore Romano* 2084 (March 4, 2009): 8.

Trocchio, Julie. "Meeting Community Needs: A Hallmark of Catholic Health Care Yesterday, Today, and Tomorrow." *Health Progress* 87, no. 3 (May-June 2006): 10-1.

Troilo, Michael Louis. "*Caritas in Veritate*, Hybrid Firms, and Institutional Arrangements." *Journal of Markets & Morality* 14, no. 1 (March 2011): 23-34.

Uelmen, Amelia J. "*Caritas in Veritate* and Chiara Lubich: Human Development from the Vantage Point of Unity." *Theological Studies* 71, no. 1 (March 2010): 29-45.

Waalkes, Scott. "Money or Business? A Case Study of Christian Virtue Ethics in Corporate Work." *Christian Scholar's Review* 38, no. 1 (September 2008): 15-40.

Wanner, Kevin J. "Prophets and Profits: On Economies of Economic Goods in Economies of Salvation." *Bulletin for the Study of Religion* 41, no. 1 (February 2012): 20-5.

Werhane, Patricia H. "Profits, Priests and Princes: Adam Smith's Emancipation of Economics from Politics and Religion." *Ethics* 106, no. 2 (January 1996): 484-5.

White, Jane K. "Not-For-Profits Versus Small Business." *Health Progress* 68, no. 7 (July 1987): 16.

White, Jane K., and John K. Iglehart. "IOM Study: Meaning for Not-For-Profits?" *Health Progress* 67, no. 10 (October 1986): 14.

PAPAL ENCYCLICALS

Benedict XVI. 2009. *Caritas in Veritate*

Benedict XVI. 2005. *Deus Caritas Est*

John Paul II. 1991. *Centesimus Annus*

John Paul II. 1987. *Sollicitudo Rei Socialis*

John Paul II. 1981. *Laborem Exercens*

Leo XIII. 1891. *Rerum Novarum*

Paul VI. 1967. *Populorum Progressio*

Pius XI. 1931. *Quadragesimo Anno*